Diabetes Friendly Recipes for the Whole Family

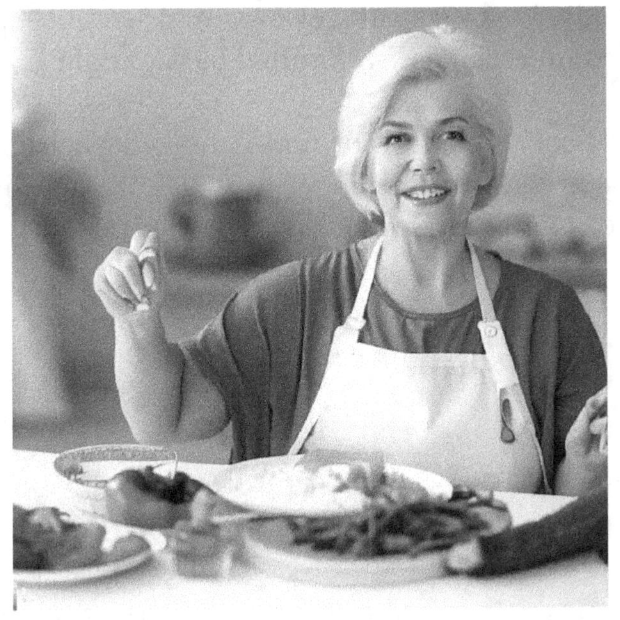

75+ Kid-Friendly Meals That Everyone Will Love

The Wellness Chef

Table of Contents

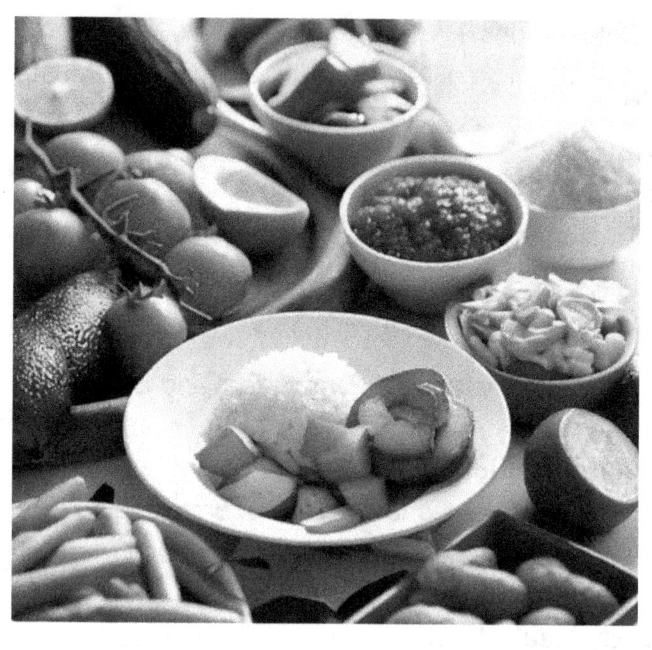

Introduction

In a world where every meal is an opportunity to nourish both body and soul, where the sizzle of a pan and the aroma of fresh ingredients dancing in harmony fill your kitchen with anticipation, we invite you on a remarkable culinary journey. Welcome to "Diabetes-Friendly Recipes for the Whole Family: 75+ Kid-Friendly Meals That Everyone Will Love."

Picture this: a family gathering around the table, laughter echoing, and a spread of delectable dishes that not only please the taste buds but also honor the wellness of every member. With each flip of the page, you're about to embark on an adventure that transcends dietary restrictions, delivering flavors that tantalize, textures that satisfy, and a bounty of healthful benefits that nourish from within.

Here, in the heart of these pages, you'll discover a treasury of recipes meticulously curated to celebrate the essence of shared meals – a collection that elevates everyday dining to a new realm of sensory delight. Our aim is not just to guide you through wholesome cooking; it's to empower you with an enchanting repertoire of dishes that are as vibrant as they are nourishing.

Dive into breakfasts that start your day with a burst of energy, savor lunches that enliven your midday pause, and indulge in dinners that transform ordinary moments into extraordinary memories. From zesty zucchini noodles to cozy apple cinnamon creations, from innovative wraps to hearty soups, from guilt-free desserts to revitalizing beverages, every recipe in this book has been thoughtfully crafted to embrace the rich tapestry of flavors while keeping blood sugar levels in check.

But this journey isn't just about the destination; it's about the joy of the process. As you read on, you'll discover insightful tips, creative techniques, and secrets to making even the pickiest of eaters fall in love with wholesome ingredients. Our goal is to infuse each mealtime with a sprinkle of enchantment, encouraging young and old to come together, share stories, and embark on a voyage of taste and togetherness.

So, whether you're a seasoned home chef or just beginning your culinary expedition, whether you're seeking ways to manage diabetes or simply eager to nourish your family with love-infused dishes, this book is your compass. Let the flavors unfold, the aromas dance, and the stories shared within these pages become an integral part of your own family narrative.

Chapter 1

Understanding Diabetes-Friendly Cooking

Welcome to a chapter that not only opens the doors to delicious possibilities but also paves the way for a healthier, more vibrant life. In "Understanding Diabetes-Friendly Cooking," we embark on a journey that not only demystifies the complexities of diabetes but also empowers you to take control of your kitchen with confidence and creativity.

Picture this: a sizzling pan, a medley of fresh produce, and the gentle aroma of herbs infusing the air. Here, cooking isn't just about nourishing the body; it's about embracing a lifestyle that celebrates flavor, balance, and well-being. And it all starts with understanding the fundamentals.

Unraveling the Diabetes Puzzle
Diabetes is more than just a medical condition; it's an intricate puzzle of blood sugar management that demands attention, care, and knowledge. In this chapter,

we'll unravel the mysteries of diabetes, helping you gain a deeper understanding of how the food you choose impacts your body's intricate dance of glucose regulation.

A Plate Full of Balance

Imagine your plate as a canvas, each dish a stroke of color that contributes to the masterpiece of your health. Here, we delve into the art of crafting balanced meals that keep your blood sugar levels steady and your taste buds delighted. From the right mix of carbohydrates to the importance of lean proteins and healthy fats, you'll learn how to assemble plates that are as visually appealing as they are nutritionally sound.

Empowering Choices, One Ingredient at a Time

The supermarket aisles might seem daunting, but armed with the right knowledge, you'll navigate them like a pro. We'll explore the world of diabetes-friendly ingredients – from the superstars that keep your energy steady to the flavor enhancers that make every bite a delight. Say goodbye to confusion and hello to informed choices that support your health goals.

Cooking, Simplified and Delightful

Cooking need not be a complicated affair. In this chapter, we'll share techniques, tips, and strategies to simplify your time in the kitchen without compromising on taste.

Whether you're a busy parent, a working professional, or an aspiring chef, these insights will transform your cooking experience into a joyous, nourishing adventure.

Connecting the Dots to Your Unique Journey
Your diabetes journey is as unique as your fingerprints. We'll guide you through understanding your body's signals, tracking your responses to different foods, and customizing your meals to suit your individual needs. Because there's no one-size-fits-all solution, but there is a world of possibilities waiting to be explored.

So, grab your apron, prepare your utensils, and let's embark on a chapter that equips you with knowledge, inspiration, and the tools to make diabetes-friendly cooking a seamless part of your life. With every dish you prepare, you're taking a step toward a healthier, more vibrant you. Let's dive in, shall we?

Embracing Balanced Meals for Wellness

Imagine your plate as a canvas of vibrant colors and diverse textures, each element harmonizing to create a masterpiece that fuels your body, nourishes your soul, and supports your overall well-being. In this chapter, we delve into the art of embracing balanced meals – a key pillar in your journey toward wellness.

The Dance of Nutrients

Balanced meals are not just about filling up a plate; they're about orchestrating a symphony of nutrients that work in harmony. Picture carbohydrates as the fuel that powers your body, proteins as the building blocks that repair and strengthen, and healthy fats as the foundation of cellular health. We'll guide you through creating a melody of these nutrients, ensuring that every bite you take contributes to your vitality.

Balancing Blood Sugar, One Bite at a Time

For those navigating the nuances of diabetes, balanced meals take on an even more significant role. By thoughtfully pairing carbohydrates with fiber, protein, and healthy fats, you can keep your blood sugar levels steady, avoiding the rollercoaster of spikes and crashes that can leave you feeling fatigued. Discover the secrets to crafting meals that leave you energized and in control.

The Plate: Your Palette of Possibilities

As you stand before your plate, imagine it as a palette awaiting your creative touch. We'll introduce you to the concept of the diabetes plate method, a visual guide that simplifies meal planning. Learn how to divide your plate into sections, allocating space for different food groups in proportions that support your health goals. Whether you're preparing a breakfast of champions or a dinner fit for royalty, this method offers flexibility and clarity.

Creating Meals that Satisfy

Balanced meals are not just about nutrients; they're about satisfaction. We'll show you how to infuse your dishes with a spectrum of flavors, textures, and colors that awaken your senses and bring joy to your table. From the crunch of fresh vegetables to the creamy allure of healthy fats, discover how to make every meal an experience to savor.

Navigating Portion Control

In a world where portion sizes can sometimes deceive, we'll equip you with the tools to navigate this tricky terrain. Portion control isn't about deprivation; it's about mindful enjoyment. Learn the art of listening to your body's signals, recognizing hunger and fullness cues, and adjusting portion sizes to match your needs.

Balanced Meals, Balanced Life
The beauty of balanced meals extends beyond the plate. It ripples into your daily life, enhancing your energy levels, supporting mental clarity, and nurturing a sense of overall well-being. With each balanced meal, you're not just nourishing your body; you're cultivating a relationship with food that's rooted in respect and care.

So, whether you're crafting breakfasts that kickstart your day, lunches that fuel your afternoon endeavors, or dinners that wind down your evenings with satisfaction, remember that balanced meals are a cornerstone of your health journey. With the knowledge gained in this chapter, you're empowered to create meals that honor your body and celebrate the joys of eating. Let's embrace the magic of balanced meals and pave the way to a life infused with vitality.

Crafting Kid-Friendly Recipes with Success

When it comes to young palates, the world of flavors and textures is an exciting playground. But let's be honest – it can also be a bit of a challenge. In this chapter, we embark on a culinary adventure tailored for the little ones in your life. Get ready to discover the art of crafting kid-friendly recipes that not only entice their taste buds but also nurture their health with every delightful bite.

Unveiling the Kid's Perspective
Ever wondered what goes on in the mind of a picky eater? It's a world where colors, shapes, and even the arrangement of food on a plate can be the difference between a joyful meal and a stubborn stand-off. We'll decode the kid's perspective, helping you understand their sensory preferences, and offering insights into how to make mealtime a win-win for everyone.

From Bland to Bold: Kid-Friendly Flavors
The world of kid-friendly flavors is far from boring. It's a realm where gentle sweetness, mild spices, and intriguing textures create a tapestry that appeals to young taste buds. We'll guide you through infusing dishes with these inviting elements, transforming mundane

ingredients into vibrant creations that kids will want to dive into.

Creative Presentation: Where Fun Meets Food

Imagine turning broccoli florets into trees, and arranging cherry tomatoes like a rainbow. Creative presentation is your secret weapon in the battle for young hearts and hungry tummies. We'll share tips and tricks to transform ordinary dishes into captivating works of art, making mealtime an adventure that sparks curiosity and joy.

Cooking Together: A Bonding Experience

Cooking isn't just about preparing food; it's a journey that families can embark on together. We'll explore the joy of involving kids in the kitchen – from choosing ingredients to mixing, measuring, and even tasting. These shared moments not only teach essential life skills but also create memories that last a lifetime.

Healthy Swaps, Happy Kids

Crafting kid-friendly recipes doesn't mean compromising on health. We'll reveal ingenious swaps that sneak in extra nutrients without compromising on taste. From incorporating hidden veggies into pasta sauces to adding a nutritional twist to familiar favorites, you'll be armed with the tools to create dishes that satisfy both taste and wellness.

A Feast for the Eyes and Palate

Kid-friendly recipes aren't just about feeding hungry stomachs; they're about stimulating young imaginations. We'll guide you through creating plates that tell stories, where a simple sandwich becomes a smiling face and a colorful fruit salad turns into a fruity jungle. By engaging their senses, you're not just feeding their bodies; you're nourishing their curiosity and creativity.

Celebrating Small Victories

In the world of kids and food, even the smallest victories are worth celebrating. A thumbs-up from a usually hesitant eater or a clean plate at the end of the meal – these are triumphs that parents and caregivers know all too well. This chapter isn't just about recipes; it's about nurturing a positive relationship with food, one bite at a time.

So, whether you're a parent, grandparent, aunt, uncle, or simply someone who loves cooking for kids, get ready to dive into the world of kid-friendly recipes with confidence and creativity. Armed with the insights and ideas from this chapter, you're about to embark on a culinary journey that fosters not only nourishment but also a love for good food that lasts a lifetime.

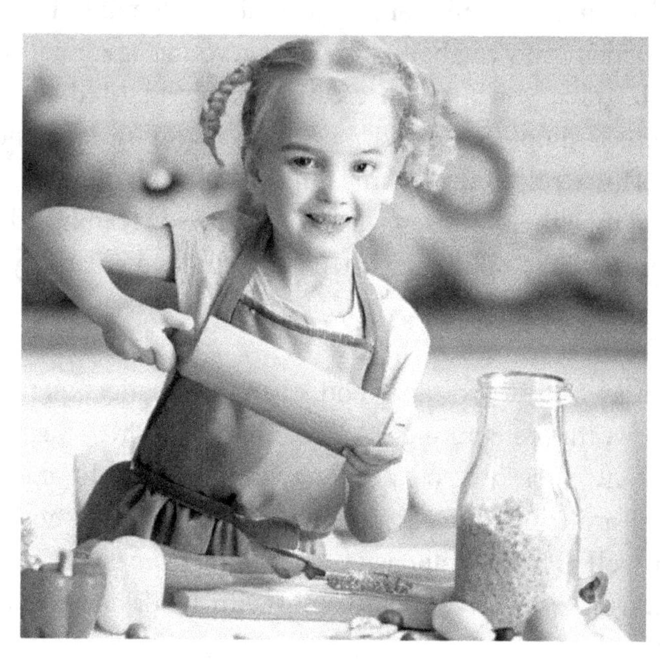

Chapter 2

Breakfast Delights

Wholesome Whole Grain Pancakes with Fresh Berries

Recipe Preparation

Get ready to awaken your taste buds with a breakfast that combines the comfort of pancakes with the goodness of whole grains and the burst of freshness from vibrant berries. These Wholesome Whole Grain Pancakes with Fresh Berries are not only a treat for your palate but also a nourishing start to your day.

Ingredients:
- 1 cup whole wheat flour
- 1 tablespoon baking powder
- 1 tablespoon honey or maple syrup
- 1 cup milk (dairy or plant-based)
- 1 egg
- 2 tablespoons melted butter or coconut oil
- 1 teaspoon vanilla extract
- A pinch of salt

- Fresh berries (such as strawberries, blueberries, or raspberries)

Instructions:

1. Mix Dry Ingredients: In a mixing bowl, combine the whole wheat flour, baking powder, and a pinch of salt. Give it a gentle whisk to ensure even distribution.

2. Create the Batter: In another bowl, whisk together the egg, milk, melted butter or coconut oil, honey or maple syrup, and vanilla extract until well combined.

3. Combine Wet and Dry: Gradually pour the wet mixture into the dry mixture while gently stirring. Mix until just combined; a few lumps are okay. Overmixing can make the pancakes tough.

4. Let It Rest: Allow the batter to rest for about 10-15 minutes. This rest time allows the flour to hydrate and results in fluffier pancakes.

5. Preheat and Grease: While the batter rests, preheat a non-stick skillet or griddle over medium heat. Lightly grease the cooking surface with a small amount of butter or oil.

6. Cooking the Pancakes: Once the skillet is hot, ladle about ¼ cup of the batter onto the skillet for each pancake. Use the back of the ladle to spread the batter into a round shape. Cook until bubbles form on the surface, and the edges look set.

7. *Flip and Finish:* Carefully flip the pancakes using a spatula, and cook for an additional 1-2 minutes until golden brown and cooked through.

8. *Serve with Fresh Berries:* Stack the cooked pancakes on a plate. Top them generously with a colorful assortment of fresh berries – strawberries, blueberries, raspberries – whatever your heart desires.

9. *Drizzle and Enjoy:* For an extra touch of sweetness, drizzle a bit more honey or maple syrup over the berry-topped pancakes. The natural sweetness of the berries combined with the gentle sweetness of the syrup creates a symphony of flavors.

10. *Dig In:* Grab your fork and knife, and dig into a stack of Wholesome Whole Grain Pancakes with Fresh Berries. Each bite is a delightful blend of the hearty pancake base and the burst of juicy, tangy berries.

Notes:
- Feel free to customize your pancakes with add-ins like chopped nuts, seeds, or even a sprinkle of cinnamon for extra flavor.

- If you're using frozen berries, thaw and drain them before topping the pancakes to prevent excess moisture.
- These pancakes are not just a breakfast option; they make for a fantastic brunch or even a wholesome dessert.

With Wholesome Whole Grain Pancakes with Fresh Berries on your plate, mornings are transformed into a celebration of flavor, health, and pure delight. This recipe is a testament to how good food can be both nourishing and indulgent, creating a perfect start to your day. Enjoy!

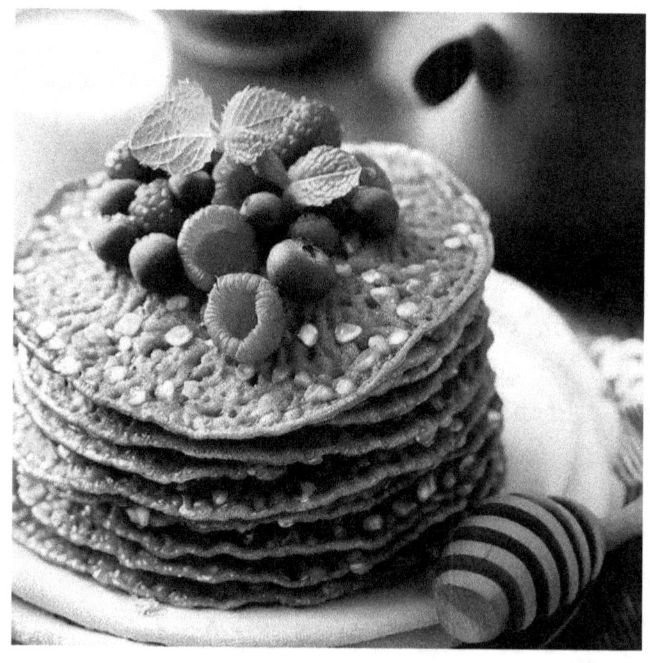

Nutrient-Rich Veggie-Packed Breakfast Burritos

Give your mornings a delicious and nutritious kickstart with these Nutrient-Rich Veggie-Packed Breakfast Burritos. Packed with a medley of colorful vegetables, protein-rich eggs, and fiber-loaded whole grains, these burritos are the perfect way to fuel your day and satisfy your taste buds.

Ingredients:
- 4 whole wheat or whole grain tortillas
- 4 large eggs
- 1 tablespoon olive oil
- 1 bell pepper, diced (use a mix of colors for visual appeal)
- 1 small red onion, diced
- 1 cup baby spinach leaves
- ½ cup black beans, drained and rinsed
- ½ cup grated cheddar cheese
- Salt and pepper to taste
- Optional toppings: salsa, avocado slices, Greek yogurt

Instructions:
1. Sauté the Veggies: In a skillet, heat the olive oil over medium heat. Add the diced bell pepper and red onion. Sauté for a few minutes until the vegetables are slightly softened and aromatic.

2. *Add the Spinach:* Stir in the baby spinach leaves and cook for another minute or two until they are wilted. Remove the skillet from heat and set aside.

3. *Scramble the Eggs:* In a bowl, whisk the eggs with a pinch of salt and pepper. Return the skillet to medium heat, push the sautéed veggies to the side, and pour in the beaten eggs. Allow them to cook undisturbed for a moment, then gently scramble until fully cooked.

4. *Assemble the Burritos:* Warm the tortillas briefly in a dry skillet or microwave. Lay them out on a clean surface. Divide the scrambled eggs, sautéed veggies, black beans, and grated cheddar cheese among the tortillas, arranging the fillings in a line down the center.

5. *Fold and Roll:* To fold the burritos, fold in the sides of the tortilla over the filling, then roll from the bottom up, tucking the sides as you go. This creates a neat, compact burrito.

6. *Optional Warm-Up:* If you prefer your burritos warm, you can lightly heat them in the skillet for a minute on each side. This step is especially helpful if you're making the burritos ahead of time.

*7. **Serve and Garnish:*** Place the prepared burritos on serving plates. If desired, top them with a dollop of Greek yogurt, slices of creamy avocado, and a spoonful of vibrant salsa.

*8. **Enjoy with Gusto:*** Grab your burrito with both hands and take a bite. Feel the satisfying crunch of fresh veggies, the creaminess of scrambled eggs, and the hearty goodness of black beans and whole grain tortillas. Each bite is a symphony of flavors and textures.

Notes:
- Feel free to customize these burritos with your favorite veggies and protein sources. Mushrooms, tomatoes, or even lean turkey sausage can make delicious additions.
- For a plant-based version, you can swap the eggs for scrambled tofu or chickpea scramble.
- Make a batch of these burritos ahead of time, wrap them in foil, and store them in the refrigerator. They make for a quick and wholesome grab-and-go breakfast on busy mornings.

With Nutrient-Rich Veggie-Packed Breakfast Burritos, your morning routine is about to get a whole lot tastier and healthier. These burritos not only provide a balanced and satisfying meal but also showcase how a little creativity in the kitchen can transform everyday ingredients into a flavorful masterpiece. So roll up your sleeves and roll up those burritos – your taste buds and your body will thank you!

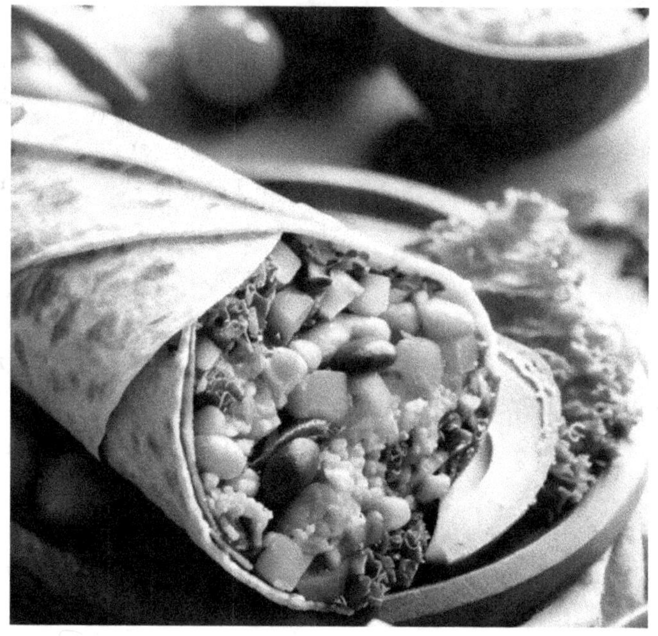

Apple Cinnamon Oatmeal Bowl for a Cozy Start

Picture a crisp morning, sunlight filtering through the curtains, and a gentle breeze that whispers promises of a new day. Now, imagine your morning routine accompanied by the comforting aroma of warm apples and cinnamon. In this recipe, we'll transport you to a world of cozy comfort with our Apple Cinnamon Oatmeal Bowl – a perfect way to start your day on a nourishing note.

Ingredients:
- 1 cup old-fashioned rolled oats
- 2 cups water or milk of your choice
- 1 apple, peeled, cored, and diced
- 1 teaspoon ground cinnamon
- 1 tablespoon honey or maple syrup (optional)
- A pinch of salt
- Toppings: chopped nuts, dried fruits, a drizzle of nut butter

Instructions:
1. In a saucepan, bring the water or milk to a gentle boil.

2. Stir in the rolled oats and a pinch of salt. Reduce the heat to a simmer and let the oats cook, stirring

occasionally, for about 5 minutes or until they reach your desired consistency.

3. While the oats are cooking, in a separate pan, sauté the diced apples with a sprinkle of cinnamon until they're soft and slightly caramelized.

4. Once the oats are cooked, remove the saucepan from the heat. Stir in the sautéed apples and the remaining ground cinnamon. If you prefer a touch of sweetness, drizzle in honey or maple syrup and give it a good stir.

5. Scoop the fragrant oatmeal into your favorite bowl.

6. Now, it's time to create your masterpiece. Sprinkle chopped nuts for a satisfying crunch, add dried fruits for bursts of sweetness, and perhaps indulge in a drizzle of nut butter for a creamy twist.

7. Take a moment to appreciate the symphony of colors, textures, and flavors before you.

8. With a spoon in hand, take that first mouthful. Let the warmth of the oatmeal and the sweetness of the apples envelop your senses. Close your eyes and savor the comforting embrace of cinnamon.

9. As you relish each bite, allow the nourishment to fuel your body and the coziness to warm your heart.

A Cozy Start, Every Morning

Our Apple Cinnamon Oatmeal Bowl isn't just a recipe; it's a ritual. It's a reminder that in a world that moves at a frenetic pace, taking a few moments for yourself and your well-being is a precious gift. With each spoonful, you're not just savoring a delicious breakfast; you're giving yourself permission to slow down, to savor life's simple pleasures, and to start your day with comfort and intention.

So, tomorrow morning, when the sun peeks over the horizon and the world awakens, treat yourself to this humble yet heartwarming bowl of Apple Cinnamon Oatmeal. Let it be your cozy companion as you step into the day, ready to embrace whatever lies ahead.

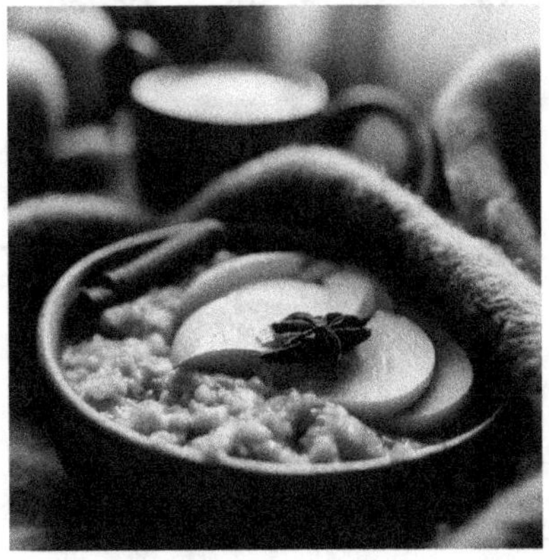

Vibrant Berry Blast Overnight Oats

Imagine waking up to a symphony of colors, a burst of flavors, and the promise of a vibrant day ahead. Our recipe for Vibrant Berry Blast Overnight Oats is more than just a breakfast; it's a delightful morning ritual that infuses your day with energy and joy from the moment you open your eyes.

Ingredients:
- 1/2 cup rolled oats
- 1/2 cup milk of your choice (dairy, almond, soy, etc.)
- 1/2 cup mixed berries (strawberries, blueberries, raspberries, etc.)
- 1 tablespoon chia seeds
- 1 teaspoon honey or maple syrup (optional)
- A dash of vanilla extract (optional)
- A pinch of salt
- Toppings: more berries, sliced bananas, nuts, and a drizzle of honey

Instructions:

1. In a jar or container, combine the rolled oats, milk, chia seeds, and a pinch of salt. If using, add the vanilla extract for an extra layer of flavor.

2. Give the mixture a good stir to ensure everything is well combined.

3. Add the mixed berries to the jar. Feel free to use a combination of your favorites – strawberries for a touch of sweetness, blueberries for antioxidants, and raspberries for a burst of tanginess.

4. If you prefer a touch of sweetness, drizzle in honey or maple syrup and gently mix.

5. Seal the jar tightly and place it in the refrigerator. Let the magic happen as the oats and chia seeds soak up the flavors overnight.

6. The next morning, as you open the refrigerator, you'll be greeted by a jar bursting with colors and anticipation.

7. Give the mixture a final stir to combine the oats, chia seeds, and berries evenly.

8. Now, it's time to make it your own. Add extra berries for a burst of freshness, sliced bananas for creamy sweetness, and a handful of nuts for satisfying crunch.

9. Take a moment to appreciate the artistry before you – a jar filled with the essence of morning vitality.

10. Grab a spoon and dig in. As each spoonful dances on your taste buds, allow the flavors to awaken your senses and the nourishment to kick-start your day.

More Than a Breakfast: A Morning Ritual

Vibrant Berry Blast Overnight Oats isn't just about starting your day; it's about embracing the potential that each morning holds. As you enjoy this colorful creation, you're nourishing your body with wholesome ingredients while celebrating the simple joys of life.

Whether you're indulging in it on a weekday rush or savoring it slowly on a leisurely weekend morning, these overnight oats are a reminder that you deserve a moment of delight and nourishment at the beginning of each day.

So, as the sun peeks over the horizon and the world awakens, treat yourself to a jar of Vibrant Berry Blast Overnight Oats. Let it be a joyful reminder that each day is an opportunity to infuse your life with color, flavor, and boundless energy.

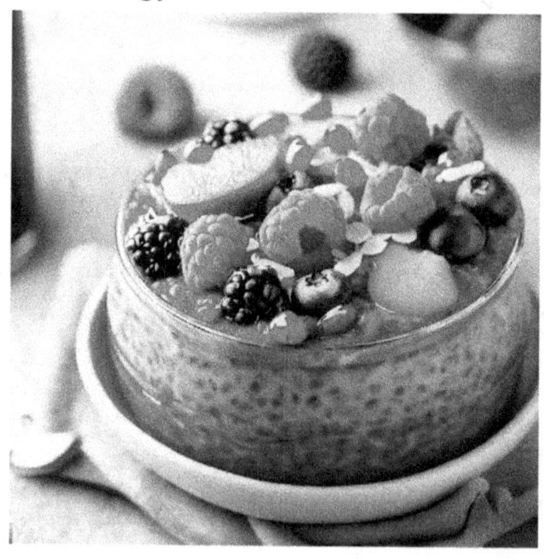

Mini Breakfast Frittatas Bursting with Flavor

In the realm of breakfast, there's something magical about dishes that are not only delicious but also delightfully convenient. Our recipe for Mini Breakfast Frittatas is a tribute to mornings made easy, without compromising on the exquisite flavors that awaken your taste buds. These bite-sized creations are the perfect canvas for your morning masterpiece.

Ingredients:
- 6 large eggs
- 1/4 cup milk of your choice (dairy, almond, etc.)
- 1/2 cup diced vegetables (bell peppers, spinach, onions, etc.)
- 1/4 cup grated cheese (cheddar, mozzarella, etc.)
- Salt and pepper to taste
- A pinch of dried herbs (thyme, oregano, etc.)
- Cooking spray or a bit of oil

Instructions:
1. Preheat your oven to 350°F (175°C). Grease a mini muffin tin with cooking spray or a touch of oil.

2. In a bowl, crack the eggs and whisk them until well beaten. Add the milk, salt, pepper, and dried herbs. Whisk again to combine.

3. Gently fold in the diced vegetables. This is where you can get creative – choose a medley of colorful veggies to make your frittatas visually appealing and bursting with flavor.

4. Pour the egg and vegetable mixture evenly into the mini muffin tin, filling each cup about two-thirds full.

5. Sprinkle the grated cheese on top of each frittata, adding a layer of gooey goodness that will melt into perfection as they bake.

6. Carefully place the muffin tin in the preheated oven and let the frittatas bake for approximately 15-18 minutes, or until they're puffed up, golden, and set in the middle.

7. As they bake, your kitchen will be filled with the tantalizing aroma of eggs, vegetables, and cheese merging into a symphony of flavor.

8. Once they're done, remove the mini frittatas from the oven and let them cool slightly in the tin before gently popping them out.

9. Arrange these bite-sized wonders on a serving platter, and let them steal the spotlight.

10. With the first bite, savor the harmony of textures and the medley of flavors that dance on your palate. The creamy eggs, the tender vegetables, and the satisfying cheese come together in a melody of morning bliss.

More Than Breakfast: A Culinary Adventure
These Mini Breakfast Frittatas are more than just a breakfast dish; they're a culinary adventure that elevates your morning routine. Whether you're enjoying them at the dining table with loved ones or grabbing a couple to go as you conquer your day, these frittatas embody the art of convenience without compromising on the quality of taste.

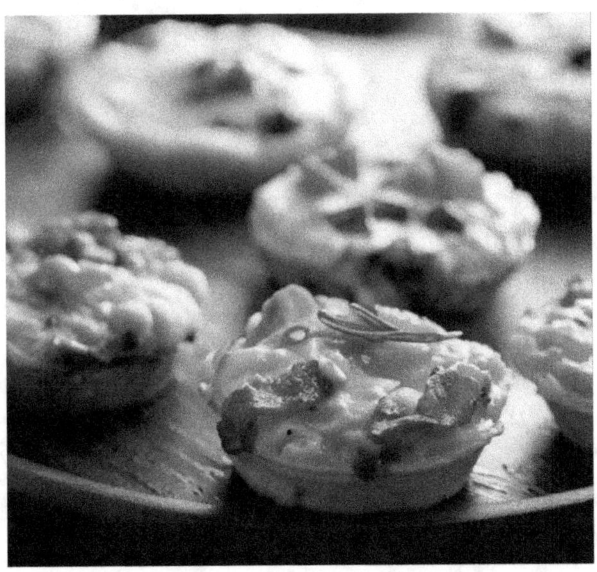

Creamy Yogurt Parfait with Crunchy Granola

Indulgence and nourishment meet in perfect harmony with our recipe for Creamy Yogurt Parfait with Crunchy Granola. Imagine a symphony of textures and flavors dancing in a glass, a delightful creation that not only tantalizes your taste buds but also pampers your senses. This parfait is a celebration of contrasts – smooth and creamy yogurt meeting the satisfying crunch of granola, all in a captivating culinary embrace.

Ingredients:
- 1 cup plain Greek yogurt
- 1/2 cup granola (homemade or store-bought)
- 1/2 cup mixed berries (strawberries, blueberries, raspberries)
- 1 tablespoon honey or maple syrup
- A drizzle of vanilla extract (optional)
- A sprinkle of chopped nuts (almonds, walnuts, etc.)
- A touch of edible flowers for a visually enchanting touch (optional)

Instructions:

1. In a bowl, mix the Greek yogurt with a drizzle of honey or maple syrup. If you desire an extra layer of flavor, add a delicate touch of vanilla extract and give it a gentle stir.

2. In a clear glass or parfait dish, begin by layering a spoonful of the creamy yogurt at the bottom. This is the canvas upon which your masterpiece will unfold.

3. Sprinkle a layer of granola on top of the yogurt. Feel the anticipation building as you create the first layer of delectable crunch.

4. Add a handful of mixed berries, letting their natural sweetness and vibrant colors add life to the parfait.

5. Repeat the layering process – yogurt, granola, berries – until you've created a visually appealing symphony of layers that beckon you to dive in.

6. On the final layer, top the parfait with a sprinkle of chopped nuts for a satisfying crunch that complements the creaminess of the yogurt.

7. For an extra touch of elegance, adorn your creation with edible flowers. Each petal is not just a visual delight; it's a reminder that food is meant to be enjoyed with all your senses.

8. As you raise the spoon to your lips, take a moment to appreciate the layers before you – a masterpiece of textures, colors, and flavors.

9. Let the first spoonful take you on a journey – the creamy yogurt enveloping your taste buds, the granola offering a satisfying bite, and the burst of berries infusing freshness into each mouthful.

Beyond Breakfast: A Sensory Delight
The Creamy Yogurt Parfait with Crunchy Granola is more than just a breakfast option; it's a sensory delight that can be enjoyed any time of day. Whether you're relishing it as a post-workout snack, savoring it as a midday treat, or presenting it as a delightful dessert, this parfait encapsulates the essence of indulgence without compromise.

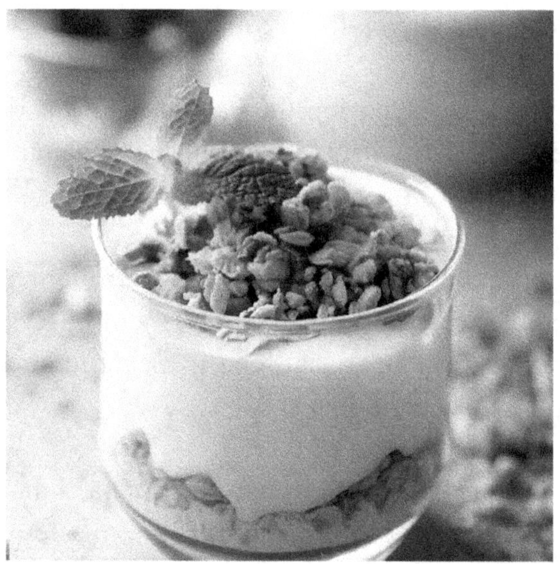

Chapter 3

Wholesome Lunches

Mini Turkey and Avocado Wraps for Satisfying Hunger

Lunchtime is a sanctuary of sustenance, a moment to refuel both body and mind. Our recipe for Mini Turkey and Avocado Wraps takes this sacred ritual to new heights, offering a balance of flavors, textures, and nourishment that promises to satisfy your hunger and elevate your midday experience.

Ingredients:
- 4 whole wheat or whole grain mini tortillas
- 8 ounces sliced turkey breast
- 1 ripe avocado, sliced
- 1 cup mixed greens (lettuce, spinach, arugula)
- 1/2 cup sliced bell peppers (red, yellow, green)
- 1/4 cup shredded carrot
- 2 tablespoons hummus or Greek yogurt spread
- Salt and pepper to taste
- A squeeze of lemon juice (optional)
- A sprinkle of dried herbs (basil, oregano, etc.)

Instructions:

1. Lay out the mini tortillas on a clean surface. These are the canvases upon which your mini wraps will come to life.

2. If using hummus or Greek yogurt spread, spread a thin layer over each tortilla. This not only adds a creamy base but also enhances the flavors that will follow.

3. Layer a generous portion of mixed greens on each tortilla. The greens not only add freshness but also provide a satisfying crunch.

4. Arrange the sliced turkey breast on top of the greens, creating a protein-packed layer that will keep you satisfied throughout the afternoon.

5. Add the sliced avocado, arranging it in a row along the center of the tortilla. Avocado brings a creamy richness that complements the lean turkey.

6. Sprinkle the sliced bell peppers and shredded carrot over the avocado. These colorful additions not only add visual appeal but also a medley of vitamins and flavors.

7. If desired, sprinkle a pinch of dried herbs over the vegetables for an aromatic touch.

8. Season the fillings with a touch of salt, pepper, and a squeeze of lemon juice for a burst of zesty brightness.

9. Begin rolling up the tortilla from one side, tucking in the fillings as you go. This will create a snug and satisfying wrap.

10. As you hold the Mini Turkey and Avocado Wrap in your hands, appreciate the layers that promise a balanced feast.

11. Take your first bite. The tender turkey meets the creamy avocado, while the crisp vegetables offer bursts of freshness. The whole wheat tortilla ties it all together in a delightful package.

A Wholesome Midday Oasis
The Mini Turkey and Avocado Wraps aren't just about appeasing your hunger; they're about transforming your lunchtime into a moment of rejuvenation. With each bite, you're not just consuming food; you're taking in a symphony of textures, a mosaic of flavors, and a plateful of nourishment.

Whether you're enjoying these wraps at your desk, savoring them on a park bench, or sharing them with loved ones around the table, these wraps encapsulate the essence of a wholesome midday oasis. They offer a reprieve from the demands of the day and an opportunity to treat yourself to a lunch that's both satisfying and revitalizing.

So, let the Mini Turkey and Avocado Wraps be your go-to companions for midday nourishment. Allow them to elevate your lunchtime routine, reminding you that every bite can be a moment of mindfulness, every wrap a symphony of satisfaction.

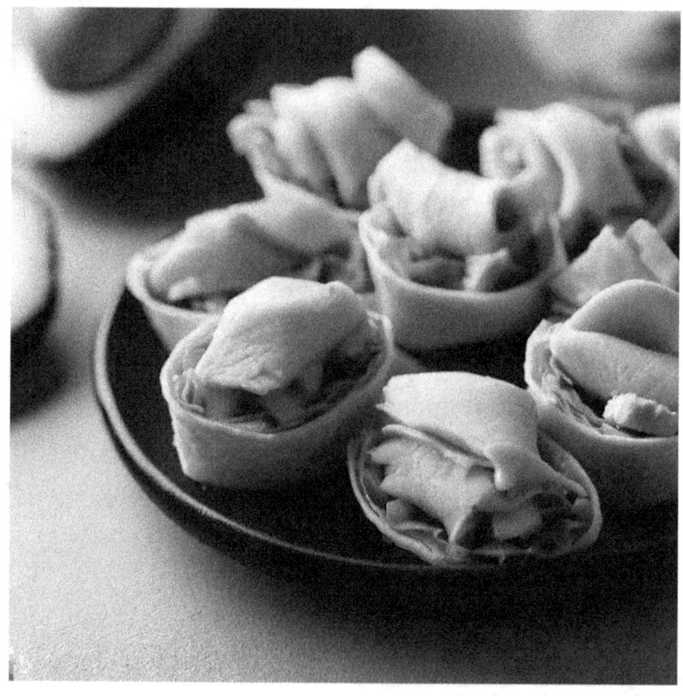

Wholesome Quinoa Salad with Roasted Veggies

In the world of culinary delights, few creations offer a symphony of flavors, colors, and nutrients quite like our Wholesome Quinoa Salad with Roasted Veggies. This recipe is a celebration of vibrant ingredients, a harmonious blend of earthy quinoa and perfectly roasted vegetables that promises to nourish your body and delight your senses.

Ingredients:
- 1 cup quinoa, rinsed and drained
- 2 cups water or vegetable broth
- 2 cups mixed vegetables (zucchini, bell peppers, cherry tomatoes, etc.)
- 2 tablespoons olive oil
- 1 teaspoon dried herbs (thyme, rosemary, etc.)
- Salt and pepper to taste
- 1/4 cup crumbled feta cheese (optional)
- 1/4 cup chopped fresh herbs (parsley, basil, etc.)
- A drizzle of balsamic glaze (optional)

Instructions:
1. Begin by preparing the quinoa. In a saucepan, combine the rinsed quinoa and water or vegetable broth. Bring it to a boil, then reduce the heat to a simmer.

Cover and let it cook for about 15 minutes or until the quinoa is fluffy and the liquid is absorbed.

2. While the quinoa cooks, preheat your oven to 400°F (200°C).

3. Prepare the mixed vegetables by cutting them into bite-sized pieces. Think of this as your canvas – a palette of colors and shapes that will make your salad visually appealing.

4. Toss the mixed vegetables with olive oil, dried herbs, salt, and pepper in a bowl. Ensure that each piece is coated with the flavorful mixture.

5. Spread the seasoned vegetables on a baking sheet in a single layer. This allows them to roast evenly and develop a delightful caramelized edge.

6. Roast the vegetables in the preheated oven for about 20-25 minutes, or until they're tender and slightly golden. The aroma that fills your kitchen will be a promise of the goodness to come.

7. Once the quinoa is cooked, fluff it with a fork and transfer it to a large mixing bowl.

8. Add the roasted vegetables to the bowl with the quinoa. Marvel at how the colors and textures come together to create a visual masterpiece.

9. If you're opting for the crumbled feta cheese, sprinkle it over the quinoa and veggies. The creamy, tangy notes of feta add depth to the dish.

10. Toss the mixture gently to combine all the elements and flavors. The quinoa acts as a canvas that soaks up the roasted vegetable goodness.

11. Just before serving, add the chopped fresh herbs for a burst of freshness and fragrance.

12. If desired, drizzle a touch of balsamic glaze over the salad. This adds a touch of sweetness and tang that elevates the flavors.

A Feast for the Senses

The Wholesome Quinoa Salad with Roasted Veggies is more than just a dish; it's a feast for your senses. As you take each forkful, you're not just experiencing a combination of tastes; you're savoring the artistry of nature's bounty and the harmony of complementary flavors.

Whether you're savoring this salad as a light lunch, a refreshing dinner, or a vibrant side dish at a gathering, it embodies the essence of wholesome nourishment. The quinoa provides a protein-packed foundation, the roasted veggies bring warmth and depth, and the fresh herbs offer a finishing touch that enlivens every bite.

So, let the Wholesome Quinoa Salad with Roasted Veggies grace your table as a reminder that good food isn't just about sustenance; it's about celebrating the vibrant medley of ingredients that nature provides. Allow it to be a testament to the beauty of simplicity, the harmony of flavors, and the joy of a meal that nourishes both body and soul.

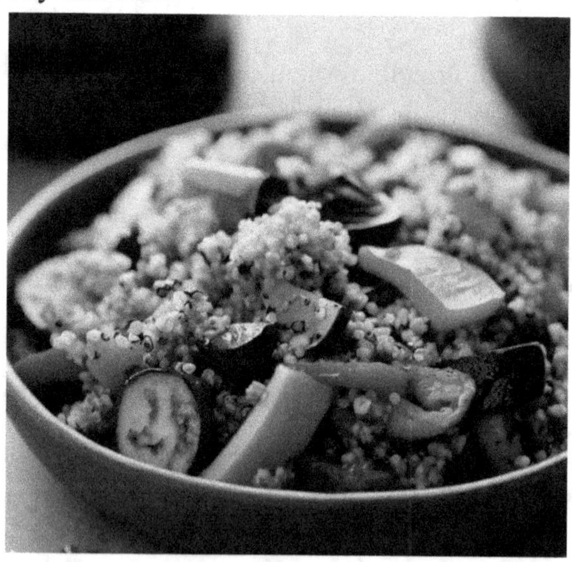

Creamy Tomato Soup with Whole Wheat Grilled Cheese Pairing

In the realm of comfort food, few combinations hold the power to evoke warmth and nostalgia quite like a steaming bowl of Creamy Tomato Soup alongside a perfectly grilled whole wheat cheese sandwich. This pairing is a testament to the simple pleasures that can turn an ordinary meal into an extraordinary experience – a harmony of textures, a fusion of flavors, and a journey that transports you to a realm of cozy contentment.

Creamy Tomato Soup:

Ingredients:
- 2 tablespoons olive oil
- 1 onion, diced
- 2 cloves garlic, minced
- 1 can (28 ounces) whole peeled tomatoes
- 2 cups vegetable or chicken broth
- 1 teaspoon dried basil
- 1/2 teaspoon dried oregano
- 1/2 cup heavy cream or coconut cream for a dairy-free option
- Salt and pepper to taste
- Fresh basil leaves for garnish (optional)

Instructions:

1. In a large pot, heat the olive oil over medium heat. Add the diced onion and minced garlic, sautéing until they're soft and fragrant.

2. Pour in the canned tomatoes (along with their juices) and the vegetable or chicken broth. Stir in the dried basil and oregano, letting the flavors meld together.

3. Bring the mixture to a gentle simmer and let it cook for about 15-20 minutes, allowing the tomatoes to break down and the flavors to intensify.

4. Using an immersion blender or a regular blender (carefully vented to release steam), blend the soup until it reaches a smooth and creamy consistency.

5. Return the soup to the pot and stir in the heavy cream, creating a lusciously creamy texture. Season with salt and pepper to taste.

6. Ladle the Creamy Tomato Soup into bowls, and if desired, garnish with fresh basil leaves for an aromatic touch.

Whole Wheat Grilled Cheese:

Ingredients:
- 4 slices of whole wheat bread
- 1 cup shredded cheese (cheddar, mozzarella, etc.)
- Butter or olive oil for grilling

Instructions:
1. Heat a skillet or griddle over medium heat.

2. Take two slices of whole wheat bread and sprinkle half of the shredded cheese on one slice of each.

3. Place the other slice of bread on top to create a sandwich.

4. Lightly butter or brush olive oil on the outside of each sandwich.

5. Place the sandwiches on the skillet or griddle and cook for a few minutes on each side, until the bread is golden and crispy and the cheese is melted.

6. Once cooked, remove the sandwiches from the heat and let them cool slightly before slicing.

Pairing: A Symphony of Comfort and Flavor

As you sit down to savor this comforting pairing, let the Creamy Tomato Soup envelop your senses with its velvety texture and the rich, robust notes of tomato and herbs. Allow the warmth of the soup to embrace you, bringing a sense of solace and familiarity to your mealtime.

Now, take a bite of the Whole Wheat Grilled Cheese – a harmonious balance of toasty bread and gooey cheese that delivers a satisfying crunch and a burst of savory goodness. The contrast between the creamy soup and the crispy sandwich creates a symphony of textures that dance on your palate.

With each spoonful of soup and every bite of grilled cheese, you're not just enjoying a meal; you're embarking on a journey that resonates with both flavor and sentiment. This pairing isn't just about nourishment; it's about creating a moment of connection, where the simple act of eating becomes an experience infused with comfort and joy.

So, let the Creamy Tomato Soup with Whole Wheat Grilled Cheese Pairing be a reminder that food has the power to evoke cherished memories and create new ones. As you savor this delightful duo, may you find solace, pleasure, and a taste of home in every mouthful.

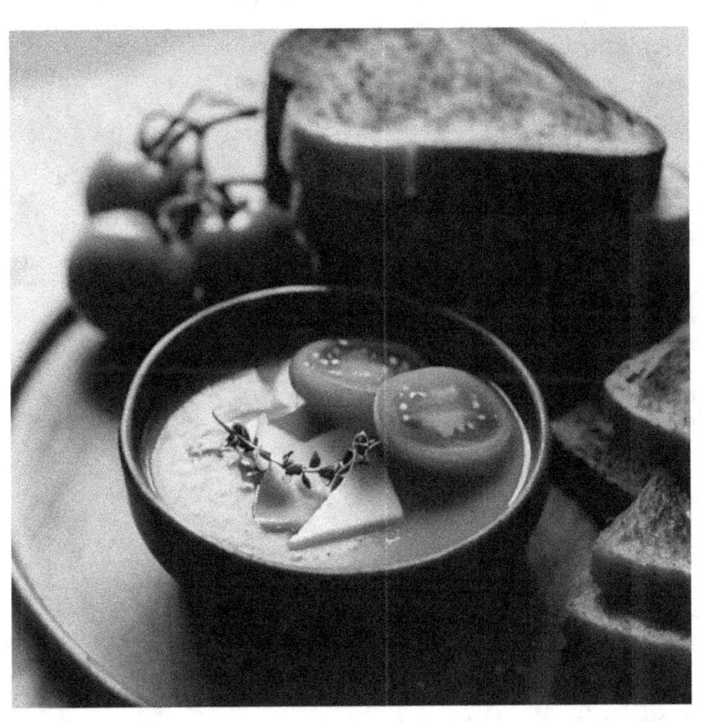

Grilled Chicken and Avocado Wraps for a Protein Boost

When the day calls for a protein-packed boost that's as satisfying as it is delicious, our Grilled Chicken and Avocado Wraps step up to the plate. This recipe is a testament to the perfect marriage of lean protein and creamy goodness, wrapped in a soft tortilla for a handheld delight that fuels your body and delights your taste buds.

Ingredients:
- 2 boneless, skinless chicken breasts
- Salt and pepper to taste
- 1 tablespoon olive oil
- 1 teaspoon paprika
- 1 teaspoon garlic powder
- 4 whole wheat or spinach tortillas
- 1 avocado, sliced
- 1 cup mixed salad greens
- 1/2 cup diced tomatoes
- 1/4 cup diced red onion
- Optional toppings: shredded cheese, Greek yogurt or sour cream, hot sauce

Instructions:
Grilled Chicken:

1. Preheat your grill or grill pan over medium-high heat.

2. Season the chicken breasts with salt, pepper, paprika, and garlic powder. Drizzle with olive oil and rub the seasonings in.

3. Place the seasoned chicken breasts on the grill and cook for about 6-7 minutes on each side, or until they're cooked through and have a nice grill marks.

4. Remove the chicken from the grill and let it rest for a few minutes before slicing it into thin strips.

Assembly:
1. Lay out the tortillas on a clean surface.

2. Divide the sliced grilled chicken evenly among the tortillas, placing the strips down the center.

3. Layer on the sliced avocado, mixed salad greens, diced tomatoes, and diced red onion.

4. If desired, sprinkle on some shredded cheese for an extra layer of indulgence.

5. Finish by drizzling a dollop of Greek yogurt or sour cream and a dash of hot sauce for a touch of zing.

6. Carefully fold in the sides of each tortilla and then roll it up tightly to create a wrap.

7. Slice each wrap in half, and marvel at the colorful medley of ingredients that await your taste buds.

Energizing Wholesomeness: A Flavorful Fusion
As you take your first bite of the Grilled Chicken and Avocado Wrap, you're met with a symphony of flavors and textures. The tender, smoky chicken pairs harmoniously with the creamy richness of avocado, while the crisp freshness of salad greens and the juicy burst of tomatoes and red onion create a medley of sensations that awaken your palate.

The protein-packed grilled chicken in these wraps not only satisfies your hunger but also provides your body with the energy it needs to conquer the day. The avocado adds a dose of healthy fats that keep you feeling full and satisfied, while the whole wheat tortilla offers a wholesome canvas that brings everything together.

Whether you're enjoying these wraps for lunch, a quick dinner, or even as a hearty snack, you're indulging in a moment of nourishment that's as delightful as it is nutritious. This recipe is a reminder that wholesome eating doesn't have to be bland or boring; it can be a mouthwatering experience that invigorates your senses and fuels your well-being.

So, let the Grilled Chicken and Avocado Wraps be your go-to solution for a protein boost that's packed with flavor and vitality. With each bite, you're not just enjoying a meal; you're embracing a fusion of taste and nourishment that energizes your body and elevates your taste experience.

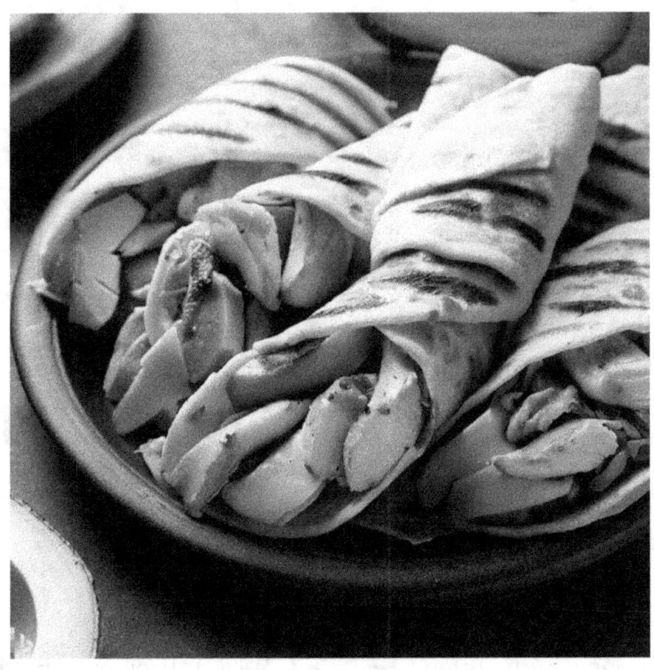

Cheesy Quinoa Stuffed Peppers Filled with Goodness

Get ready to embark on a culinary adventure that marries vibrant flavors, wholesome ingredients, and a touch of cheesy indulgence. Our recipe for Cheesy Quinoa Stuffed Peppers is a celebration of colors, textures, and the joy of savoring a dish that's as delightful to your taste buds as it is nourishing to your body. Each bite is a journey into a world where goodness resides within the embrace of a pepper.

Ingredients:
- 4 large bell peppers (red, yellow, or orange)
- 1 cup cooked quinoa
- 1 cup black beans (canned or cooked)
- 1 cup diced vegetables (zucchini, corn, tomatoes, etc.)
- 1 cup grated cheese (cheddar, mozzarella, etc.)
- 1 teaspoon olive oil
- 1 teaspoon chili powder
- 1/2 teaspoon cumin
- Salt and pepper to taste
- Fresh cilantro or parsley for garnish

Instructions:
1. Preheat your oven to 375°F (190°C). Prepare a baking dish by lightly greasing it with olive oil.

2. Cut the tops off the bell peppers and remove the seeds and membranes from inside. Create a hollow space for the stuffing, ensuring that the peppers can stand upright.

3. In a pan, heat the olive oil over medium heat. Add the diced vegetables and sauté until they're tender and slightly caramelized.

4. Stir in the cooked quinoa, black beans, chili powder, cumin, salt, and pepper. Let the flavors meld together for a few minutes.

5. Remove the pan from the heat and stir in half of the grated cheese, allowing it to melt and coat the quinoa mixture with its delicious creaminess.

6. Carefully spoon the quinoa mixture into the hollowed bell peppers, pressing down gently to pack in the goodness.

7. Sprinkle the remaining grated cheese on top of each stuffed pepper, letting it create a golden crust as it bakes.

8. Place the stuffed peppers in the prepared baking dish and pop them into the preheated oven. Let them bake for about 20-25 minutes, or until the peppers are tender and the cheese is bubbly and golden.

9. As the peppers bake, your kitchen will be enveloped in the irresistible aroma of cheesy quinoa mingling with the rich essence of peppers.

10. Once they're done, carefully remove the stuffed peppers from the oven and let them cool slightly.

11. Garnish with fresh cilantro or parsley, adding a burst of vibrant color and a touch of herbal freshness to the dish.

12. With a sense of anticipation, cut into the stuffed pepper, revealing the layers of goodness within.

A Fiesta of Flavors and Nutrients
Cheesy Quinoa Stuffed Peppers are more than just a meal; they're a culinary fiesta that celebrates the beauty of nourishing ingredients. With every bite, you experience the hearty combination of protein-packed quinoa, fiber-rich black beans, and a medley of vegetables that burst with vitamins and minerals.

The cheesy topping is not just a treat for your taste buds; it's a symbol of how indulgence and health can coexist in perfect harmony. Each mouthful is a tribute to the culinary artistry that can turn simple ingredients into a symphony of flavors and textures.

So, whether you're savoring these stuffed peppers as a satisfying dinner, presenting them as an impressive dish for guests, or simply enjoying the pleasure of cooking with love, let Cheesy Quinoa Stuffed Peppers be your reminder that every bite you take can be a celebration of goodness, both on your plate and in your life.

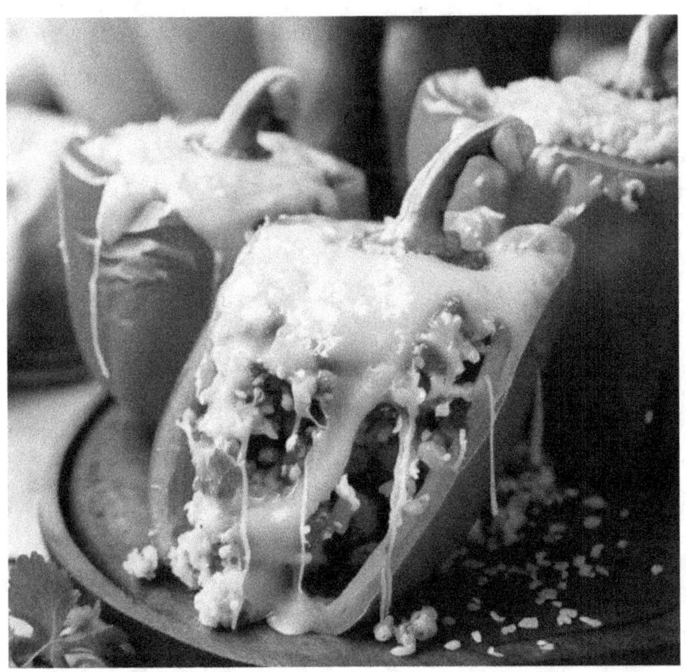

Turkey and Veggie Pinwheels to Delight

Imagine a snack that's not only delicious but also a burst of wholesome goodness. Our recipe for Turkey and Veggie Pinwheels is a creation that fuses convenience, nutrition, and flavor into delightful bites that are perfect for any occasion. These pinwheels are a testament to the art of snacking smartly without compromising on taste.

Ingredients:
- Whole wheat tortillas or wraps
- Sliced turkey (or your choice of protein)
- Hummus or cream cheese spread
- Sliced vegetables (bell peppers, cucumbers, carrots, etc.)
- A handful of spinach leaves
- Salt, pepper, and your favorite herbs for seasoning

Instructions:
1. Lay out the whole wheat tortillas or wraps on a clean surface.

2. Spread a thin layer of hummus or cream cheese over each tortilla. This not only adds a creamy touch but also helps hold the pinwheels together.

3. Layer the sliced turkey evenly over the spread, covering the tortilla from edge to edge.

4. Arrange the sliced vegetables on top of the turkey. Choose a variety of colors for visual appeal and a range of nutrients.

5. Sprinkle a touch of salt, pepper, and your favorite herbs over the vegetables. This adds a burst of flavor that complements the freshness of the ingredients.

6. Lay a handful of spinach leaves on top of the vegetables, adding an extra layer of texture and nutrition.

7. Carefully roll up the tortilla into a tight cylinder, ensuring that the fillings stay intact.

8. With a sharp knife, slice the rolled tortilla into individual pinwheels. Each slice is a bite-sized package of goodness waiting to be savored.

9. Arrange the pinwheels on a serving platter, letting the colorful layers create an enticing visual display.

10. Whether you're serving these pinwheels at a gathering, enjoying them as a midday snack, or packing them for on-the-go nourishment, let each bite remind you of the art of mindful eating.

Beyond Snacking: A Nutritious Adventure

Turkey and Veggie Pinwheels are more than just a snack; they're a journey into a world where nutrition and flavor collide. With every bite, you're treating your taste buds to the rich, savory goodness of turkey, the crisp freshness of vegetables, and the creamy delight of hummus or cream cheese.

But these pinwheels are more than just ingredients; they're a reminder that snacking can be a celebration of health and a demonstration of self-care. By choosing whole wheat tortillas, lean protein, and a medley of colorful vegetables, you're making a conscious choice to nourish your body with every nibble.

So, whether you're indulging in these pinwheels as a satisfying snack, sharing them with loved ones, or simply enjoying the pleasure of eating with intention, let Turkey and Veggie Pinwheels be a part of your journey toward a life where every bite you take is a step toward delight and well-being.

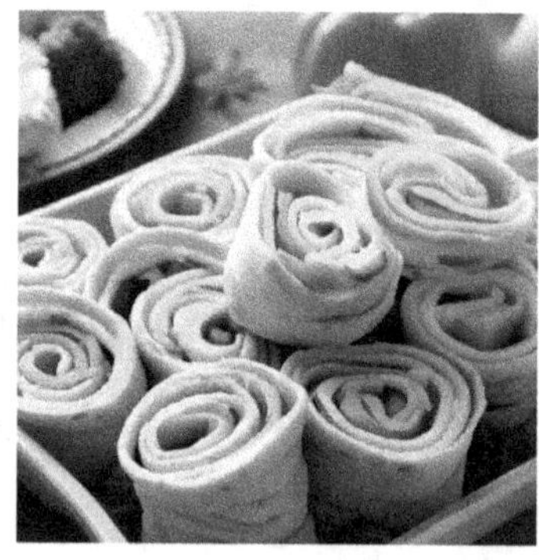

Chapter 4

Sides and Accompaniments

Roasted Garlic Mashed Cauliflower for Comfort

In the realm of dining, side dishes are more than just accompaniments; they're supporting characters that elevate a meal to a symphony of flavors. Our recipe for Roasted Garlic Mashed Cauliflower is a tribute to the art of creating sides that not only complement the main course but also stand as stars in their own right. Get ready to experience the comfort of mashed potatoes with a nutritious twist that's sure to delight your taste buds.

Ingredients:
- 1 head of cauliflower, chopped into florets
- 3-4 garlic cloves, peeled
- 1 tablespoon olive oil
- Salt and pepper to taste
- 1/4 cup plain Greek yogurt
- Fresh herbs for garnish (parsley, chives, etc.)

Instructions:

1. Preheat your oven to 400°F (200°C).

2. In a bowl, toss the cauliflower florets and peeled garlic cloves with olive oil, salt, and pepper. Ensure that the vegetables are well coated with the oil and seasonings.

3. Spread the cauliflower and garlic on a baking sheet in a single layer. Roast them in the preheated oven for about 20-25 minutes, or until they're tender and slightly golden.

4. As the cauliflower and garlic roast, your kitchen will be enveloped in the irresistible aroma of garlic mingling with the earthy essence of cauliflower.

5. Once they're done roasting, remove the baking sheet from the oven and let the vegetables cool slightly.

6. Transfer the roasted cauliflower and garlic to a food processor. Add the Greek yogurt, which lends a creamy touch without the need for excessive butter or cream.

7. Blend the mixture until it reaches a smooth and creamy consistency. You're creating a cauliflower puree that's a testament to how simple ingredients can be transformed into culinary magic.

8. Taste and adjust the seasoning, adding more salt or pepper if needed.

9. With a spoon, scoop the Roasted Garlic Mashed Cauliflower into a serving bowl, ready to take its place on your dining table.

10. Garnish with fresh herbs – a sprinkle of parsley or chives adds a burst of color and an herbal aroma that complements the dish.

11. With the first spoonful, experience the comforting embrace of mashed cauliflower that's creamy, savory, and infused with the warmth of roasted garlic.

Comfort with a Nutritional Twist
Roasted Garlic Mashed Cauliflower is more than just a side dish; it's a celebration of comfort food with a nutritional twist. As you savor each spoonful, you're not just indulging in a creamy delight; you're treating your body to the vitamins, minerals, and fiber-rich goodness that cauliflower brings.

This side dish is a reminder that comfort need not come at the cost of health. With a clever blend of roasted vegetables and the creaminess of Greek yogurt, you're creating a dish that nourishes your soul while honoring your well-being.

So, whether you're pairing Roasted Garlic Mashed Cauliflower with a hearty main course, serving it as a side at a gathering, or simply enjoying it as a solo indulgence, let it remind you that the art of side dishes lies in their ability to offer both comfort and nourishment, one delectable bite at a time.

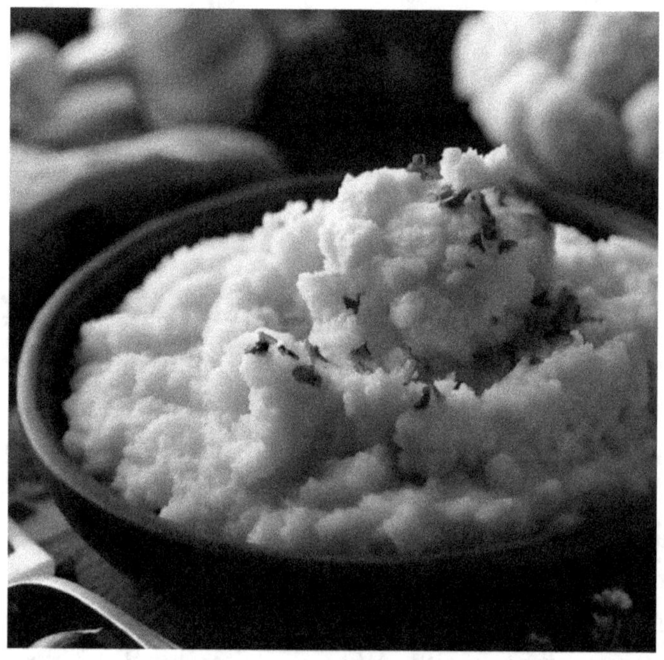

Colorful Quinoa Salad for Vibrancy

In the realm of salads, there's one that stands out not only for its wholesome ingredients but also for its vibrant array of colors. Our recipe for Colorful Quinoa Salad is a celebration of nature's palette, where fresh vegetables, hearty quinoa, and zesty dressing come together to create a symphony of flavors and a feast for the eyes. Get ready to experience a salad that's not only nourishing but also a work of culinary art.

Ingredients:
- 1 cup cooked quinoa (white, red, or a mix)
- 1 cup diced mixed vegetables (bell peppers, cherry tomatoes, cucumbers, red onions, etc.)
- 1/2 cup chopped fresh herbs (parsley, mint, cilantro)
- 1/4 cup crumbled feta cheese (optional)
- 1/4 cup chopped nuts (walnuts, almonds, etc.)
- Zest and juice of a lemon
- 2 tablespoons olive oil
- Salt and pepper to taste

Instructions:
1. In a large bowl, combine the cooked quinoa with the diced mixed vegetables. Choose an array of colors for visual vibrancy and a variety of nutrients.

2. Toss in the chopped fresh herbs, letting their aromatic essence infuse the salad with freshness and depth of flavor.

3. If you're including crumbled feta cheese, sprinkle it over the quinoa and vegetables. Its creamy tanginess will add a delightful contrast to the textures and flavors.

4. Add the chopped nuts to the bowl. Their satisfying crunch will create a harmonious balance with the tender quinoa and vegetables.

5. In a separate small bowl, whisk together the lemon zest, lemon juice, olive oil, salt, and pepper. This zesty dressing will bring a burst of citrusy brightness to the salad.

6. Drizzle the dressing over the quinoa mixture, ensuring that every ingredient is coated in its zesty embrace.

7. Gently toss the salad to combine all the elements, letting the flavors meld together and the colors create a visual spectacle.

8. With a sense of anticipation, transfer the Colorful Quinoa Salad to a serving platter or individual bowls.

9. As you take the first bite, experience the medley of flavors that come together in a harmonious dance. The nutty quinoa, the juicy vegetables, the tangy feta, and the zesty dressing create a celebration of taste and texture.

A Feast for the Senses and Health
Colorful Quinoa Salad is more than just a salad; it's a sensory experience that celebrates the beauty of nature's bounty. With every forkful, you're treating yourself to a combination of textures, colors, and flavors that nourish not only your body but also your spirit.

This salad is a reminder that food can be both nutritious and a delight to the senses. The combination of fresh vegetables, protein-packed quinoa, and zesty dressing is a testament to how a thoughtful composition of ingredients can transform a simple dish into a culinary masterpiece.

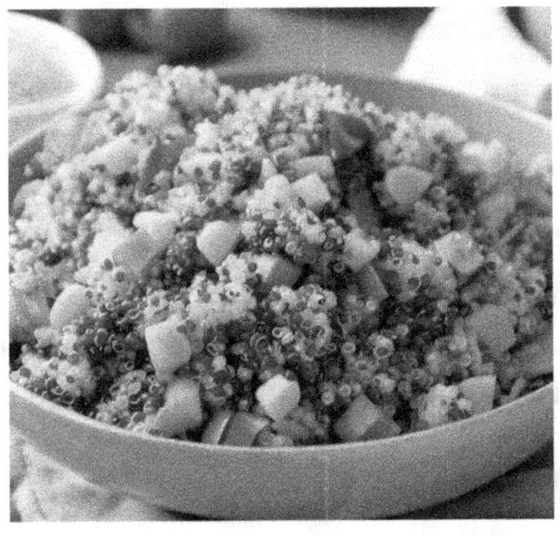

Sautéed Spinach with Garlic and Zesty Lemon Twist

In the world of leafy greens, there's a dish that's not only quick and easy but also bursts with flavor and vitality. Our recipe for Sautéed Spinach with Garlic and Zesty Lemon Twist is a celebration of simplicity, where a handful of ingredients come together to create a dish that's as delightful to your taste buds as it is nourishing to your body. Get ready to experience a symphony of flavors that elevates spinach to a whole new level.

Ingredients:
- Fresh spinach leaves, washed and dried
- 2-3 garlic cloves, minced
- Zest and juice of a lemon
- Olive oil for sautéing
- Salt and pepper to taste
- A pinch of red pepper flakes (optional)

Instructions:

1. In a large skillet, heat a drizzle of olive oil over medium heat.

2. Add the minced garlic to the skillet and let it sizzle gently, infusing the oil with its aromatic essence.

3. Carefully add the fresh spinach leaves to the skillet. They may initially seem voluminous, but spinach wilts quickly, so don't be discouraged by the abundance.

4. Using tongs or a spatula, gently toss the spinach in the skillet. The heat will start to wilt the leaves, reducing their volume and concentrating their flavor.

5. As the spinach wilts, sprinkle a touch of salt, pepper, and, if you desire a bit of heat, a pinch of red pepper flakes. These seasonings will complement the earthy notes of spinach and the garlicky aroma.

6. Continue tossing the spinach until it's uniformly wilted and coated with the garlic-infused oil and seasonings.

7. Remove the skillet from the heat. Add the zest and juice of a lemon, letting the citrusy brightness envelop the spinach in a zesty embrace.

8. Gently toss the spinach once more, ensuring that the lemon zest and juice are evenly distributed.

9. With anticipation, transfer the Sautéed Spinach with Garlic and Zesty Lemon Twist to a serving dish.

10. As you take the first forkful, experience the medley of flavors dancing on your palate. The tender spinach leaves, the rich undertones of garlic, and the zesty burst of lemon create a green delight that's both invigorating and comforting.

A Wholesome Culinary Experience

Sautéed Spinach with Garlic and Zesty Lemon Twist is more than just a side dish; it's a culinary experience that proves that simplicity can be a gateway to extraordinary flavors. With each bite, you're not just enjoying a handful of spinach; you're indulging in a symphony of taste sensations that awaken your senses.

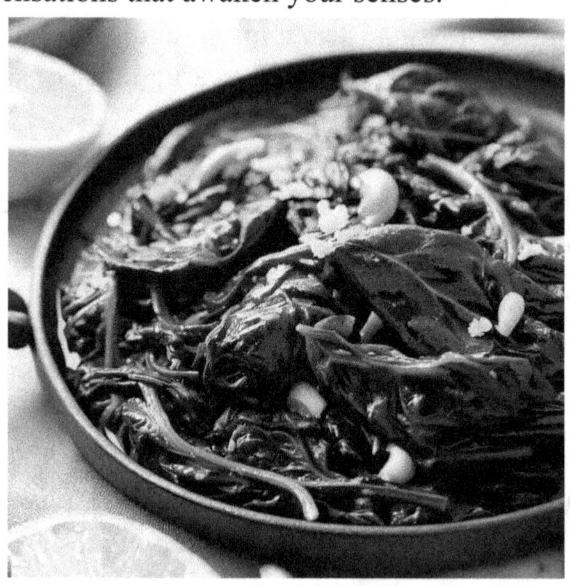

Chapter 5

Delicious Dinners

Baked Herb-Crusted Chicken Tenders for Wholesome Crunch

In the realm of dinners that satisfy both the palate and the need for nourishment, there's a recipe that combines crispy indulgence with wholesome goodness. Our creation of Baked Herb-Crusted Chicken Tenders is a tribute to the art of crafting meals that not only delight your taste buds but also nourish your body. Get ready to experience a dish that elevates chicken tenders to a new level of flavor and crunch, all while keeping things nutritious.

Ingredients:
- Chicken tenders or boneless, skinless chicken breasts, cut into strips
- Whole wheat breadcrumbs or panko breadcrumbs
- Fresh herbs (thyme, rosemary, parsley, etc.), finely chopped
- Parmesan cheese, grated (optional)
- Olive oil or cooking spray
- Salt and pepper to taste

- Greek yogurt or dijon mustard for dipping (optional)

Instructions:

1. Preheat your oven to 400°F (200°C). Prepare a baking sheet by lining it with parchment paper or lightly greasing it with olive oil.

2. In a bowl, mix the breadcrumbs, chopped fresh herbs, and grated Parmesan cheese if using. This mixture will be the flavorful and crunchy coating for your chicken tenders.

3. Season the chicken tenders with a sprinkle of salt and pepper.

4. Dip each chicken tender into the breadcrumb mixture, pressing gently to ensure the coating adheres evenly to the chicken.

5. Place the coated chicken tenders on the prepared baking sheet. Make sure they're spaced apart so they can cook evenly and become delightfully crispy.

6. Drizzle a bit of olive oil over the coated chicken tenders or give them a light spray with cooking spray. This will help them achieve that golden crunch in the oven.

7. Bake the chicken tenders in the preheated oven for about 15-20 minutes, or until they're cooked through and the coating is crispy and golden.

8. As they bake, your kitchen will be filled with the irresistible aroma of herbs and chicken mingling together in a symphony of flavor.

9. Once they're done, remove the chicken tenders from the oven and let them cool slightly.

10. With a sense of anticipation, transfer the Baked Herb-Crusted Chicken Tenders to a serving platter, ready to be enjoyed.

11. For an extra touch of flavor, serve these tenders with a dipping sauce made from Greek yogurt or dijon mustard. This adds a creamy or tangy contrast that complements the crispy coating.

12. As you take the first bite, experience the medley of textures – the satisfying crunch of the herb-infused coating giving way to the tender, succulent chicken within.

Crispy and Nutritious Culinary Adventure
Baked Herb-Crusted Chicken Tenders are more than just a dinner; they're a culinary adventure that proves you

don't have to compromise on taste to enjoy a wholesome meal. With each bite, you're treating yourself to the savory embrace of fresh herbs, the satisfying crunch of the coating, and the protein-rich goodness of chicken.

This dish is a reminder that indulgence can coexist with nutrition. By baking instead of frying, and by using whole wheat breadcrumbs and fresh herbs, you're creating a meal that's both satisfying and good for you.

So, whether you're serving Baked Herb-Crusted Chicken Tenders as a main course, presenting them as a crowd-pleasing dish at gatherings, or simply enjoying them as a comfort food that ticks all the boxes, let them be a reminder that culinary excellence lies in the balance between flavor and nourishment.

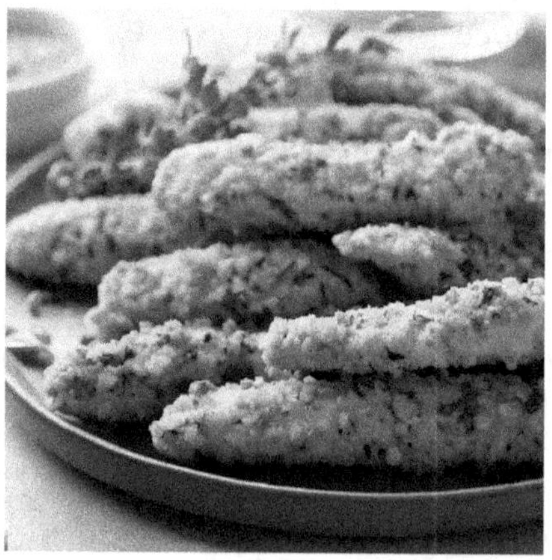

Zucchini Noodles with Lean Turkey Meatballs for a Twist

Dive into a dinner that brings together the best of both worlds — a twist on traditional comfort paired with the goodness of wholesome ingredients. Our recipe for Zucchini Noodles with Lean Turkey Meatballs is a celebration of culinary innovation, where tender zucchini noodles embrace lean turkey meatballs in a symphony of flavors and textures that redefine the concept of a satisfying meal.

Ingredients:
For the Turkey Meatballs:
- Lean ground turkey
- Whole wheat breadcrumbs
- Egg
- Chopped fresh herbs (parsley, basil, oregano)
- Garlic powder
- Salt and pepper

For the Zucchini Noodles:
- Zucchini, spiralized into noodles
- Olive oil
- Garlic, minced
- Crushed red pepper flakes (optional)
- Salt and pepper

For the Tomato Sauce:
- Crushed tomatoes or tomato sauce
- Chopped fresh basil
- Garlic, minced
- Olive oil
- Salt and pepper

Instructions:

For the Turkey Meatballs:
1. Preheat your oven to 375°F (190°C). Line a baking sheet with parchment paper.

2. In a bowl, combine the ground turkey, whole wheat breadcrumbs, egg, chopped fresh herbs, garlic powder, salt, and pepper. Mix gently until the ingredients are well incorporated.

3. Shape the mixture into small meatballs and place them on the prepared baking sheet.

4. Bake the turkey meatballs in the preheated oven for about 20-25 minutes, or until they're cooked through and nicely browned.

For the Zucchini Noodles:
1. In a skillet, heat a drizzle of olive oil over medium heat.

2. Add the minced garlic and optional crushed red pepper flakes to the skillet. Sauté for a minute until fragrant.

3. Add the spiralized zucchini noodles to the skillet. Sauté them for a few minutes until they're tender but still have a slight crunch.

4. Season the zucchini noodles with salt and pepper, then remove them from the heat.

For the Tomato Sauce:
1. In a separate saucepan, heat a bit of olive oil over medium heat.

2. Add the minced garlic and sauté until aromatic.

3. Pour in the crushed tomatoes or tomato sauce and let it simmer for a few minutes.

4. Stir in the chopped fresh basil and season the sauce with salt and pepper to taste.

Bringing It All Together:
1. Serve the zucchini noodles on a plate, topped with a generous ladle of the tomato sauce.

2. Nestle the lean turkey meatballs on the bed of zucchini noodles, letting them settle comfortably into their flavorful embrace.

3. As you take your first forkful, experience the medley of flavors – the zesty tomato sauce, the tender zucchini noodles, and the herb-infused turkey meatballs – all coming together in a harmonious dance of innovation and satisfaction.

A Fusion of Comfort and Health

Zucchini Noodles with Lean Turkey Meatballs is more than just a meal; it's a fusion of comfort and health that illustrates the beauty of culinary exploration. With every bite, you're not just enjoying a classic combination; you're indulging in a medley of textures and flavors that nourish both body and soul.

This dish is a reminder that traditional comfort foods can be reimagined in ways that elevate taste and nutrition. By using zucchini noodles instead of traditional pasta and lean turkey instead of beef, you're creating a meal that's both familiar and refreshing.

So, whether you're relishing Zucchini Noodles with Lean Turkey Meatballs as a satisfying dinner, sharing it with loved ones, or simply enjoying the thrill of creating a twist on the ordinary, let it remind you that the joy of cooking lies in the balance between innovation and tradition.

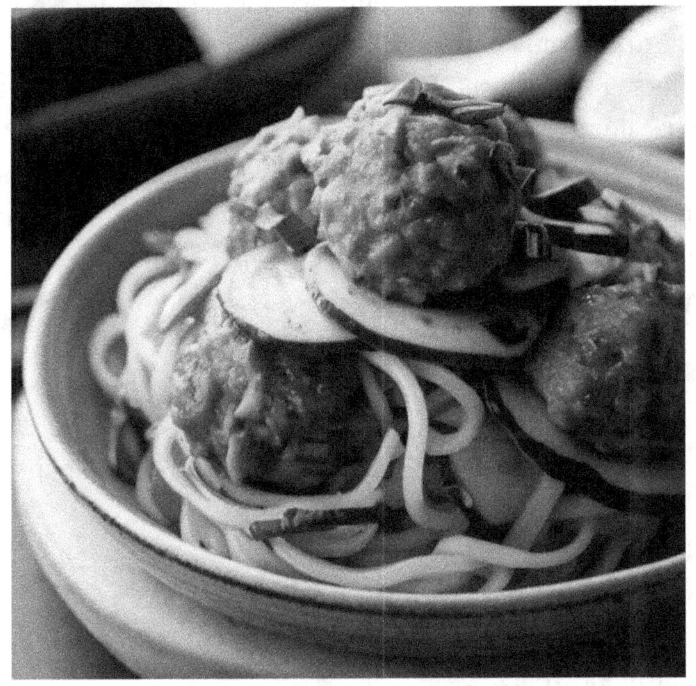

Fish Tacos with Refreshing Mango Salsa

Prepare to embark on a culinary journey that transports you to the sunny shores of coastal flavors and the vibrant colors of a fiesta. Our recipe for Fish Tacos with Refreshing Mango Salsa is a celebration of taste and texture, where tender fish meets the zing of mango salsa in a symphony that captures the essence of a seaside feast. Get ready to experience a dish that's not only a treat for your taste buds but also a feast for your senses.

Ingredients:
For the Fish:
- Fresh white fish fillets (such as cod, tilapia, or mahi-mahi)
- Olive oil
- Ground cumin
- Smoked paprika
- Garlic powder
- Salt and pepper

For the Mango Salsa:
- Ripe mango, diced
- Red onion, finely chopped
- Red bell pepper, diced
- Fresh cilantro, chopped
- Jalapeño, finely chopped (optional)
- Lime juice
- Salt and pepper

For Assembling:
- Soft corn or flour tortillas
- Shredded lettuce or cabbage
- Sour cream or Greek yogurt
- Lime wedges

Instructions:
For the Fish:
1. Preheat a grill or stovetop pan over medium-high heat.

2. Drizzle the fish fillets with olive oil and sprinkle with ground cumin, smoked paprika, garlic powder, salt, and pepper. These seasonings will infuse the fish with a burst of smoky flavor.

3. Grill the fish fillets for a few minutes on each side, or until they're cooked through and flaky. Cooking time will depend on the thickness of the fillets.

4. Once done, remove the fish from the grill or pan and let it rest briefly before flaking it into bite-sized pieces.

For the Mango Salsa:
1. In a bowl, combine the diced mango, finely chopped red onion, diced red bell pepper, chopped fresh cilantro, and optional jalapeño for a touch of heat.

2. Drizzle the lime juice over the ingredients and sprinkle with salt and pepper. The citrusy zing of lime will add a refreshing contrast to the sweetness of the mango.

3. Gently toss the ingredients to ensure they're well mixed, letting the colors and flavors intermingle.

Assembling the Tacos:
1. Warm the soft tortillas in a dry skillet or over an open flame until they're pliable and slightly toasted.

2. Lay out the warmed tortillas and layer each one with a generous spoonful of the flaked fish.

3. Top the fish with a portion of the refreshing mango salsa, letting the vibrant colors create an inviting display.

4. Add a handful of shredded lettuce or cabbage for a crunchy textural element.

5. Drizzle with a dollop of sour cream or Greek yogurt for a creamy touch.

6. Squeeze a wedge of lime over each taco, adding a burst of citrusy brightness.

7. With a sense of anticipation, fold the tortillas and enjoy the explosion of flavors and textures in each bite.

A Seaside Feast at Home
Fish Tacos with Refreshing Mango Salsa are more than just a meal; they're a culinary adventure that brings the essence of the coast to your own kitchen. With each bite, you're transported to the world of seaside flavors, where tender fish meets the sweet and tangy allure of mango salsa.

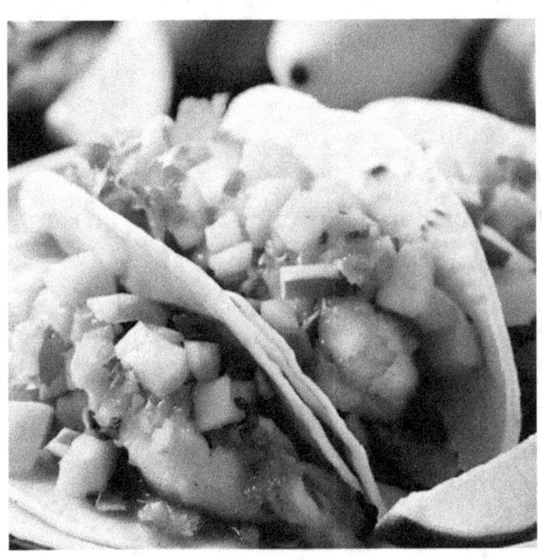

Teriyaki Tofu Stir-Fry for Plant-Powered Goodness

Step into a world where plant-based ingredients take center stage in a dish that's as satisfying as it is nourishing. Our Teriyaki Tofu Stir-Fry is a celebration of plant-powered goodness, where tender tofu dances alongside vibrant vegetables in a symphony of flavors that redefine what it means to indulge in a wholesome meal. Get ready to experience a dish that not only delights your taste buds but also fuels your body with the power of nature's bounty.

Ingredients:

- Firm tofu, cubed
- Assorted vegetables (bell peppers, broccoli, carrots, snap peas, etc.), sliced or chopped
- Teriyaki sauce (store-bought or homemade)
- Low-sodium soy sauce or tamari
- Garlic, minced
- Ginger, grated
- Sesame oil
- Sesame seeds for garnish (optional)
- Cooked brown rice or quinoa for serving

Instructions:

1. Begin by pressing the cubed tofu to remove excess moisture. You can do this by wrapping the tofu in a clean

kitchen towel or paper towels and gently pressing down. This helps the tofu absorb the flavors of the stir-fry sauce better.

2. In a bowl, whisk together the teriyaki sauce, low-sodium soy sauce or tamari, minced garlic, grated ginger, and a drizzle of sesame oil. This mixture will be the flavorful marinade for the tofu.

3. Place the cubed tofu in the marinade and let it soak for at least 15-20 minutes, allowing the flavors to infuse into the tofu.

4. In a large skillet or wok, heat a bit of sesame oil over medium-high heat.

5. Add the marinated tofu to the skillet, letting it sizzle and cook until it's golden and slightly crispy on the outside.

6. Once the tofu is cooked to your liking, transfer it to a plate and set it aside.

7. In the same skillet, add a touch more sesame oil if needed. Toss in the sliced or chopped vegetables and stir-fry them until they're tender yet still crisp.

8. Return the cooked tofu to the skillet with the vegetables, creating a colorful medley of plant-powered goodness.

9. Pour the remaining teriyaki sauce over the tofu and vegetables, ensuring that everything is coated in the savory and slightly sweet flavors of the sauce.

10. Gently toss the stir-fry to combine all the elements and let the flavors meld together.

11. With anticipation, serve the Teriyaki Tofu Stir-Fry over cooked brown rice or quinoa, allowing the nutty grains to soak up the delectable sauce.

12. If desired, sprinkle sesame seeds over the dish for a touch of crunch and visual appeal.

A Plant-Powered Symphony of Taste
Teriyaki Tofu Stir-Fry is more than just a meal; it's a symphony of tastes and textures that showcases the artistry of plant-based cooking. With every bite, you're not just enjoying a stir-fry; you're experiencing the harmony of tender tofu, crisp vegetables, and the bold flavors of teriyaki.

This dish is a reminder that plant-based eating is not only good for your body but also a feast for your senses. The combination of protein-packed tofu, nutrient-rich vegetables, and umami-rich teriyaki sauce is a testament to how nature's bounty can create culinary magic.

So, whether you're savoring Teriyaki Tofu Stir-Fry as a nourishing dinner, sharing it with friends and family, or simply celebrating the joy of plant-powered cooking, let it be a reminder that flavor, nourishment, and delight can all be found in the embrace of nature's finest ingredients.

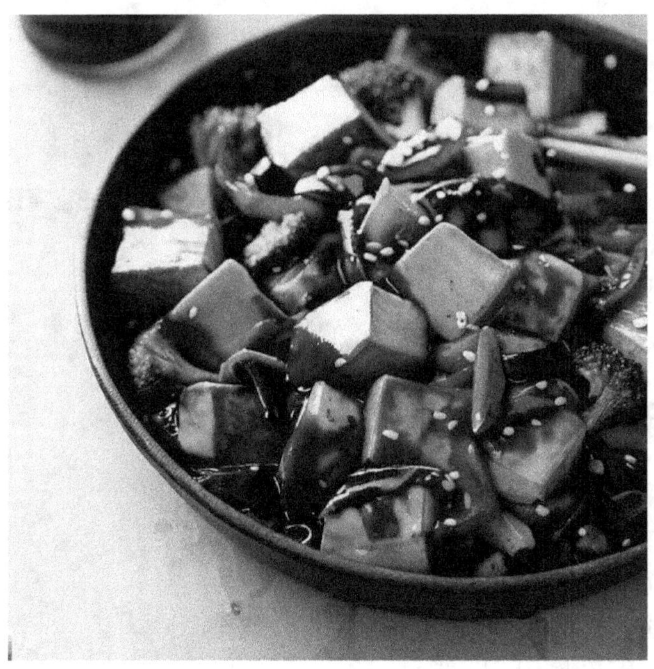

Veggie-Packed Spaghetti Bolognese for Wholesome Indulgence

Get ready to savor a comforting classic that's been reinvented with a wholesome twist. Our recipe for Veggie-Packed Spaghetti Bolognese is a celebration of heartiness and health, where the rich flavors of Bolognese sauce meld with an abundance of colorful vegetables to create a dish that satisfies both your cravings and your body's needs. Prepare to experience a plate of goodness that's as nourishing as it is indulgent.

Ingredients:

- Whole wheat spaghetti or your choice of pasta
- Lean ground meat (beef, turkey, chicken, or plant-based option)
- Onion, finely chopped
- Carrot, finely chopped
- Celery, finely chopped
- Bell peppers, diced
- Zucchini, diced
- Garlic, minced
- Crushed tomatoes
- Tomato paste
- Fresh basil and oregano, chopped
- Red wine (optional)
- Olive oil
- Salt and pepper

- Grated Parmesan cheese (optional)

Instructions:

1. In a large pot, heat a drizzle of olive oil over medium heat. Add the chopped onion, carrot, and celery, sautéing until they're softened and aromatic.

2. Add the diced bell peppers and zucchini to the pot, letting their vibrant colors brighten up the mixture.

3. Stir in the minced garlic, allowing its fragrance to infuse the vegetables.

4. If using ground meat, add it to the pot and cook until it's browned and cooked through. If opting for a plant-based version, add your choice of plant-based protein.

5. Pour in the crushed tomatoes and tomato paste, creating the rich and hearty base of the Bolognese sauce.

6. If you're using red wine, add a splash to the pot. This optional step adds depth and complexity to the sauce.

7. Sprinkle in the chopped fresh basil and oregano, letting their herbal essence infuse the sauce with flavor.

8. Season the sauce with salt and pepper to taste. Let it simmer gently for about 20-30 minutes, allowing the flavors to meld and develop.

9. As the sauce simmers, prepare the whole wheat spaghetti or pasta of your choice according to the package instructions.

10. Once the pasta is cooked, drain it and toss it with a drizzle of olive oil to prevent sticking.

11. Serve the Veggie-Packed Bolognese sauce over the cooked pasta. For an extra touch, sprinkle with grated Parmesan cheese.

12. As you take your first forkful, experience the harmony of flavors – the rich and savory Bolognese sauce merging with the sweetness of vegetables and the satisfying texture of whole wheat pasta.

Balancing Comfort and Nutrition

Veggie-Packed Spaghetti Bolognese is more than just a meal; it's a testament to the art of finding balance between comfort and nutrition. With every forkful, you're not just indulging in a classic dish; you're treating yourself to the wholesome embrace of colorful vegetables, lean protein, and nourishing whole wheat pasta.

This dish is a reminder that traditional comfort foods can be transformed into nutritional powerhouses without sacrificing taste. By incorporating an array of vegetables into the sauce and opting for whole wheat pasta, you're creating a plate that's as satisfying to your body as it is to your cravings.

So, whether you're savoring Veggie-Packed Spaghetti Bolognese as a cozy dinner, sharing it with loved ones, or simply relishing the joy of a balanced indulgence, let it remind you that the pleasure of dining lies in the ability to nourish both your appetite and your well-being.

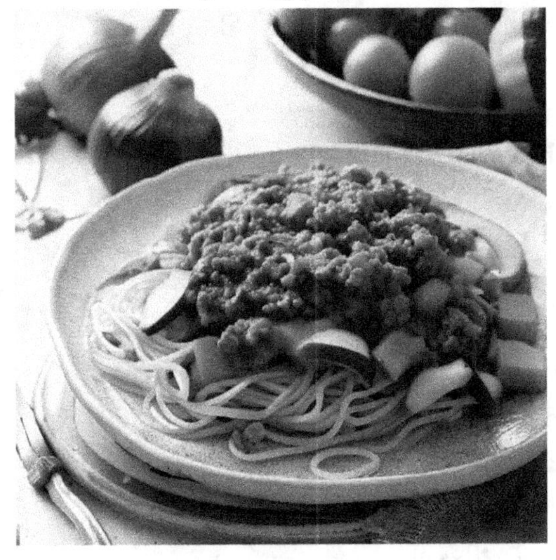

Lemon Herb Grilled Salmon with Roasted Garden Vegetables

Elevate your dining experience with a harmonious medley of nature's finest offerings. Our recipe for Lemon Herb Grilled Salmon with Roasted Garden Vegetables is a celebration of simplicity and sophistication, where succulent salmon meets the vibrant essence of garden-fresh vegetables. Get ready to embark on a culinary journey that transports you to a garden oasis of taste and nourishment.

Ingredients:
For the Lemon Herb Grilled Salmon:
- Fresh salmon fillets
- Lemon zest and juice
- Fresh herbs (rosemary, thyme, dill)
- Garlic, minced
- Olive oil
- Salt and pepper

For the Roasted Garden Vegetables:
- Assorted garden vegetables (zucchini, bell peppers, cherry tomatoes, red onion)
- Olive oil
- Balsamic vinegar
- Fresh herbs (basil, oregano)
- Salt and pepper

Instructions:

For the Lemon Herb Grilled Salmon:

1. In a bowl, whisk together lemon zest, lemon juice, minced garlic, chopped fresh herbs, olive oil, salt, and pepper. This fragrant marinade will infuse the salmon with a burst of citrusy and herbal delight.

2. Place the salmon fillets in a shallow dish and pour the marinade over them. Let them marinate for about 20-30 minutes, allowing the flavors to permeate the fish.

3. Preheat your grill to medium-high heat. Brush the grates with a bit of oil to prevent sticking.

4. Place the marinated salmon fillets on the grill, skin-side down. Grill for a few minutes on each side, or until the salmon is cooked to your desired level of doneness and has those beautiful grill marks.

5. As the salmon grills, your senses will be treated to the tantalizing aroma of lemon and herbs mingling with the smokiness of the grill.

For the Roasted Garden Vegetables:

1. Preheat your oven to 400°F (200°C).

2. Chop the assorted garden vegetables into bite-sized pieces. This array of colors and textures will bring a garden-fresh symphony to your plate.

3. In a bowl, toss the chopped vegetables with olive oil, balsamic vinegar, chopped fresh herbs, salt, and pepper. Ensure the vegetables are evenly coated with the oil and seasonings.

4. Spread the coated vegetables on a baking sheet in a single layer. Roast them in the preheated oven for about 20-25 minutes, or until they're tender and slightly caramelized.

Bringing It All Together:
1. Arrange the Lemon Herb Grilled Salmon fillets on a serving platter, their glistening surface a testament to the vibrant marinade.

2. Surround the salmon with a generous portion of the roasted garden vegetables, letting their jewel-like colors create a visually captivating display.

3. With a sense of anticipation, take your first forkful, experiencing the delicate flakiness of the salmon complemented by the zesty brightness of lemon and herbs, all harmonizing with the comforting sweetness of the roasted vegetables.

A Symphony of Taste and Wellness

Lemon Herb Grilled Salmon with Roasted Garden Vegetables is more than just a meal; it's a symphony of flavors and nourishment that celebrates the beauty of fresh, wholesome ingredients. With every bite, you're immersing yourself in a composition of textures, aromas, and tastes that awaken both your palate and your spirit.

This dish is a reminder that the finest culinary pleasures often stem from the simplest of ingredients. By combining the elegance of grilled salmon with the vibrant vitality of garden vegetables, you're creating a plate that speaks of both indulgence and wellness.

So, whether you're savoring this masterpiece as a centerpiece of a dinner gathering, relishing it as a solo indulgence, or simply embracing the joy of preparing a meal that nourishes both body and soul, let it remind you that the art of cooking lies in the ability to create a symphony of taste that resonates deeply with every forkful.

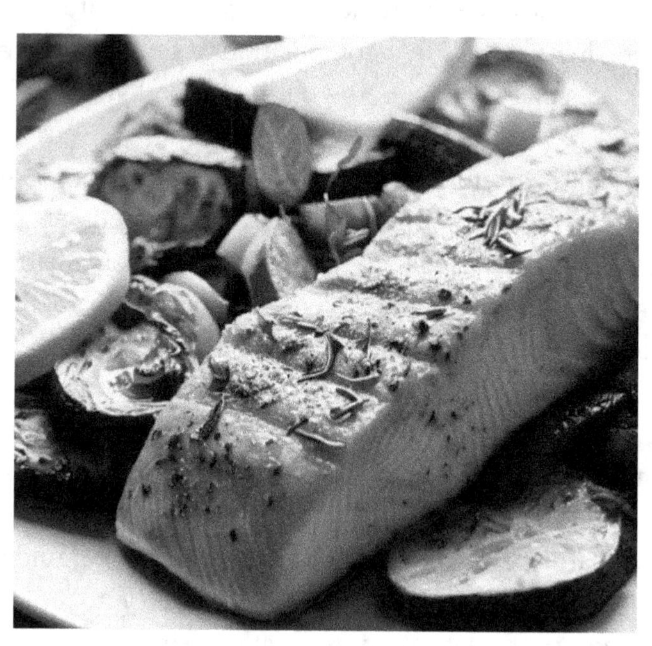

Chapter 6

Snack Time Favorites

Crunchy Chickpea Snack Mix for Nourishing Crunch

When the urge for a satisfying snack strikes, there's a delightful mix that combines crunchiness with wholesome goodness. Our recipe for Crunchy Chickpea Snack Mix is a celebration of flavor and texture, where roasted chickpeas mingle with an array of ingredients to create a snack that's as delightful to your taste buds as it is nourishing to your body. Get ready to experience a medley of tastes that redefine snack time.

Ingredients:
- Canned chickpeas, drained and rinsed
- Olive oil
- Your choice of seasonings (smoked paprika, cumin, chili powder, etc.)
- Salt and pepper
- Mixed nuts (almonds, cashews, etc.)
- Dried cranberries or raisins
- Roasted seeds (pumpkin, sunflower, etc.)
- Optional: a pinch of cayenne pepper for a kick

Instructions:

1. Preheat your oven to 400°F (200°C).

2. Pat the canned chickpeas dry with a clean kitchen towel or paper towels. Removing excess moisture will help them become extra crispy when roasted.

3. In a bowl, toss the chickpeas with olive oil, your choice of seasonings, salt, and pepper. The seasonings will infuse the chickpeas with layers of flavor.

4. Spread the seasoned chickpeas on a baking sheet in a single layer. Roast them in the preheated oven for about 20-25 minutes, or until they're golden brown and crispy. Shake the baking sheet a few times during roasting to ensure even cooking.

5. Once the chickpeas are roasted to perfection, remove them from the oven and let them cool slightly.

6. In a separate bowl, combine mixed nuts, dried cranberries or raisins, and roasted seeds. This mixture will add an array of textures and flavors to the snack mix.

7. Add the roasted chickpeas to the nut and seed mixture. If you desire a touch of heat, sprinkle a pinch of cayenne pepper over the mix.

8. Gently toss all the ingredients together to ensure an even distribution of flavors and textures.

9. Portion the Crunchy Chickpea Snack Mix into small bowls or resealable bags, ready to be enjoyed whenever your snack cravings strike.

10. As you take your first handful, experience the medley of tastes – the satisfying crunch of chickpeas, the richness of nuts, the sweetness of dried cranberries, and the earthiness of roasted seeds.

A Wholesome Snack Adventure
Crunchy Chickpea Snack Mix is more than just a snack; it's a journey of flavors and textures that elevates snacking to a new level of satisfaction. With each bite, you're not just appeasing your cravings; you're treating yourself to a nourishing blend of ingredients that fuel both your body and your taste buds.

This mix is a reminder that snacking can be a conscious choice that offers both indulgence and nutrition. By combining protein-packed chickpeas with nutrient-rich nuts, seeds, and dried fruits, you're creating a snack that's as satisfying as it is healthful.

So, whether you're enjoying Crunchy Chickpea Snack Mix as a midday treat, sharing it with friends, or simply appreciating the joy of a snack that satisfies on every level, let it be a reminder that even in the realm of snacking, you have the power to create moments of nourishment and delight.

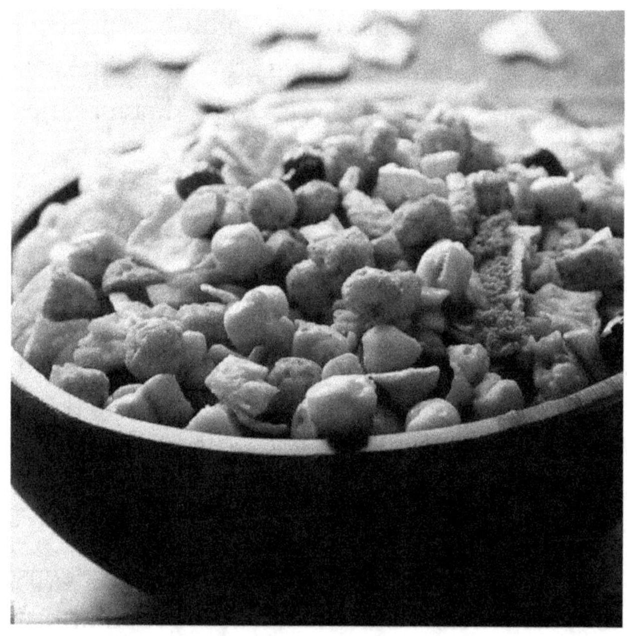

Greek Yogurt Parfait with Mixed Berries for Creamy Delight

Prepare to indulge in a dessert that's as luscious as it is wholesome, as creamy as it is refreshing. Our recipe for Greek Yogurt Parfait with Mixed Berries is a celebration of contrasts – the velvety smoothness of Greek yogurt paired with the burst of sweetness from a medley of mixed berries. Get ready to experience a dessert that's not only a treat for your taste buds but also a celebration of nourishing decadence.

Ingredients:
- Greek yogurt, plain or vanilla-flavored
- Mixed berries (such as strawberries, blueberries, raspberries, and blackberries)
- Honey or maple syrup
- Granola or chopped nuts for crunch (optional)
- Fresh mint leaves for garnish (optional)

Instructions:
1. Begin by washing and preparing the mixed berries. If using strawberries, remove the stems and slice them for easier layering.

2. In a bowl, drizzle a bit of honey or maple syrup over the mixed berries. Toss them gently to coat the berries in a touch of sweetness.

3. In serving glasses or bowls, layer the Greek yogurt with the mixed berries. Begin with a dollop of Greek yogurt, followed by a layer of mixed berries. Repeat this layering process until you have a beautiful symphony of yogurt and berries.

4. For an added layer of texture and flavor, sprinkle granola or chopped nuts between the layers. This will provide a delightful crunch that contrasts with the creamy yogurt and juicy berries.

5. Drizzle a bit more honey or maple syrup over the top layer of berries for a finishing touch of sweetness.

6. If you're feeling particularly artistic, garnish your parfaits with a few fresh mint leaves. Their vibrant green color adds a touch of elegance and freshness.

7. As you take your first spoonful, experience the harmony of flavors and textures – the velvety richness of Greek yogurt mingling with the natural sweetness of the mixed berries.

A Treat for the Senses and Well-Being

Greek Yogurt Parfait with Mixed Berries is more than just a dessert; it's a symphony of taste and wellness that reminds us that indulgence can also be nourishing. With every spoonful, you're not just enjoying the creaminess of yogurt and the sweetness of berries; you're giving your body a gift of vitamins, antioxidants, and probiotics.

This parfait is a reminder that dessert can be a delightful intersection of pleasure and health. By combining creamy Greek yogurt with nature's bounty of fresh berries, you're creating a dessert that's not only satisfying but also good for you.

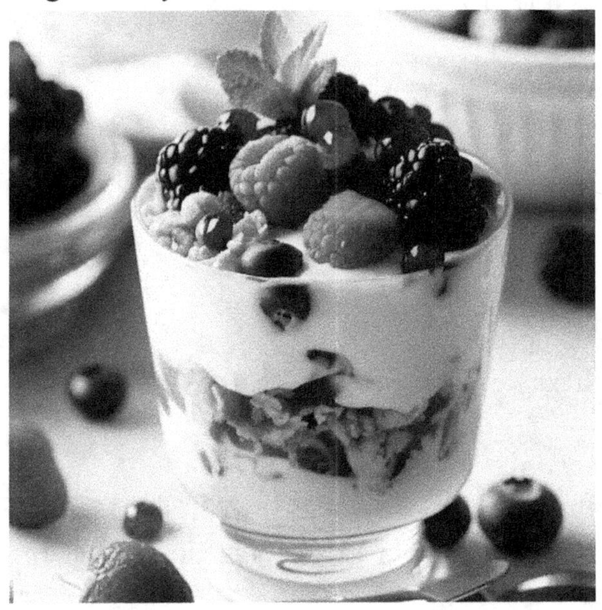

Oven-Baked Sweet Potato Fries for Guilt-Free Snacking

Indulge your cravings without compromise as you dive into a snacking sensation that's both satisfying and nourishing. Our recipe for Oven-Baked Sweet Potato Fries brings you the perfect balance of flavor and health, where the humble sweet potato is transformed into crispy, golden goodness that's hard to resist. Prepare to savor a guilt-free treat that's as delightful to your taste buds as it is to your well-being.

Ingredients:
- Sweet potatoes, peeled and cut into fries
- Olive oil
- Paprika
- Garlic powder
- Ground cumin
- Salt and pepper
- Fresh parsley, chopped (optional)

Instructions:

1. Preheat your oven to 425°F (220°C). Line a baking sheet with parchment paper to prevent sticking.

2. In a bowl, toss the sweet potato fries with a drizzle of olive oil, ensuring they're coated evenly. The olive oil will help the fries crisp up beautifully in the oven.

3. Sprinkle the sweet potato fries with paprika, garlic powder, ground cumin, salt, and pepper. These seasonings will infuse the fries with a medley of flavors.

4. Spread the seasoned sweet potato fries on the prepared baking sheet in a single layer, allowing space between each fry for even baking.

5. Bake the fries in the preheated oven for about 20-25 minutes, flipping them halfway through. Keep an eye on them to achieve the perfect balance between crispiness and tenderness.

6. Once they're golden and crispy, remove the sweet potato fries from the oven and let them cool slightly.

7. Transfer the Oven-Baked Sweet Potato Fries to a serving dish, ready to be enjoyed.

8. For an extra touch of freshness, sprinkle the chopped fresh parsley over the fries.

A Healthful Twist on Classic Comfort
Oven-Baked Sweet Potato Fries are more than just a snack; they're a testament to the art of transforming simple ingredients into a satisfying delight. With every bite, you're not just munching on fries; you're savoring

the natural sweetness of sweet potatoes mingling with a symphony of spices.

This dish is a reminder that snacking can be both enjoyable and healthful. By baking instead of deep-frying, and by using nutrient-rich sweet potatoes, you're creating a guilt-free indulgence that's kind to your taste buds and your body.

So, whether you're relishing Oven-Baked Sweet Potato Fries as a savory side, serving them as a crowd-pleasing appetizer, or simply enjoying the thrill of guilt-free snacking, let them be a reminder that the joy of eating lies in the ability to savor every bite without compromise.

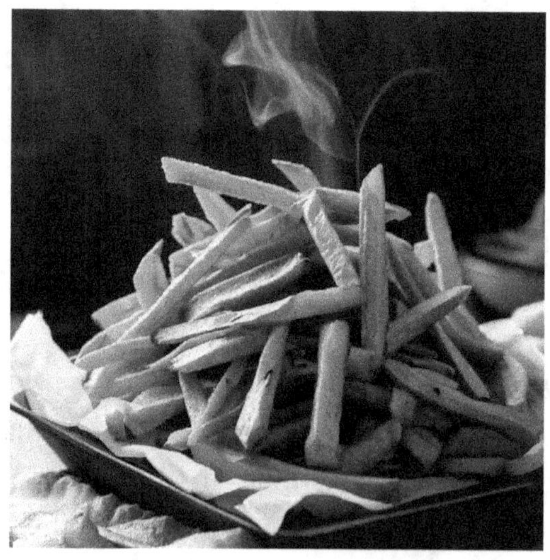

Chapter 7

Creative Sides

Rainbow Veggie Skewers with Creamy Hummus Dip

Elevate your side dish game with a burst of color and flavor that's as appealing to the eyes as it is to the palate. Our recipe for Rainbow Veggie Skewers with Creamy Hummus Dip is a celebration of vibrant vegetables paired with a luscious hummus that creates a medley of taste sensations. Get ready to embark on a culinary journey where each skewer is a work of art and every dip is a creamy delight.

Ingredients:
For the Rainbow Veggie Skewers:
- A colorful variety of vegetables (bell peppers, cherry tomatoes, zucchini, red onion, etc.), chopped into bite-sized pieces
- Olive oil
- Fresh herbs (rosemary, thyme, etc.), chopped (optional)
- Salt and pepper
- Wooden skewers, soaked in water if necessary

For the Creamy Hummus Dip:
- Prepared hummus (store-bought or homemade)
- Lemon juice
- Olive oil
- Garlic, minced
- Salt and pepper
- Paprika and fresh parsley for garnish (optional)

Instructions:
For the Rainbow Veggie Skewers:
1. Preheat a grill or stovetop grill pan over medium-high heat.

2. In a bowl, toss the chopped vegetables with a drizzle of olive oil, chopped fresh herbs if using, salt, and pepper. The olive oil and herbs will enhance the natural flavors of the vegetables.

3. Thread the colorful vegetable pieces onto the wooden skewers, creating a rainbow pattern that's as visually pleasing as it is delicious.

4. Grill the vegetable skewers for a few minutes on each side, or until they're charred and tender. Cooking time will vary depending on the vegetables and your desired level of doneness.

5. Once grilled to perfection, remove the skewers from the grill and let them rest for a moment.

For the Creamy Hummus Dip:
1. In a bowl, combine the prepared hummus, a squeeze of lemon juice, a drizzle of olive oil, minced garlic, salt, and pepper. Mix well until the ingredients are smoothly blended.

2. Taste and adjust the seasonings to your preference, adding more lemon juice or salt if needed.

3. If desired, garnish the hummus with a sprinkle of paprika and fresh parsley for an extra pop of color and flavor.

Bringing It All Together:
1. Arrange the Rainbow Veggie Skewers on a serving platter, letting their vibrant colors create a striking display.

2. Place a bowl of the Creamy Hummus Dip in the center of the platter, ready to accompany the colorful skewers.

3. As you take your first skewer and dip it into the luscious hummus, experience the harmonious marriage of textures – the crispness of grilled vegetables meeting the creaminess of the hummus.

A Visual Feast for the Senses

Rainbow Veggie Skewers with Creamy Hummus Dip is more than just a side; it's a feast for the senses that celebrates both taste and aesthetics. With every bite, you're not just enjoying a snack; you're savoring a burst of flavors that comes alive in a palette of colors.

This dish is a reminder that creative sides can be as enjoyable to make as they are to consume. By combining the visual appeal of a rainbow of vegetables with the creamy satisfaction of hummus, you're crafting an appetizing masterpiece that's as nourishing as it is beautiful.

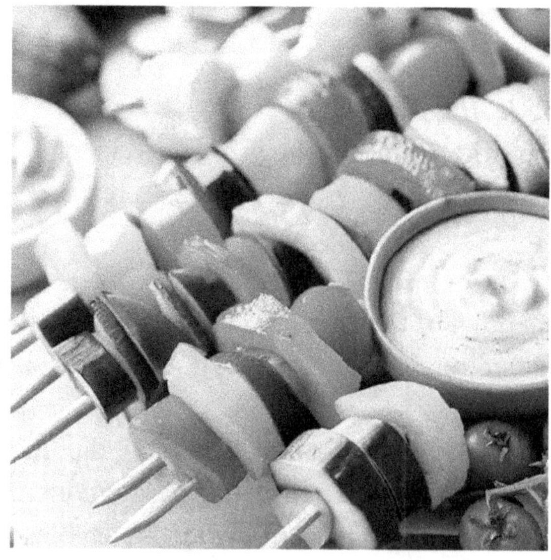

Fragrant Garlic and Herb Quinoa Pilaf

Embark on a culinary journey that infuses nourishing grains with the aromatic richness of garlic and a symphony of fresh herbs. Our recipe for Fragrant Garlic and Herb Quinoa Pilaf is a celebration of wholesome goodness and vibrant taste, where quinoa takes center stage and is transformed into a fragrant masterpiece. Get ready to savor a dish that not only satisfies your appetite but also awakens your senses.

Ingredients:
- Quinoa, rinsed and drained
- Olive oil
- Garlic, minced
- Fresh herbs (such as thyme, rosemary, and parsley), chopped
- Vegetable or chicken broth
- Salt and pepper
- Lemon zest (optional)
- Toasted nuts or seeds for garnish (optional)

Instructions:
1. In a saucepan, heat a drizzle of olive oil over medium heat. Add the minced garlic and sauté until it's fragrant and just beginning to turn golden.

2. Add the rinsed quinoa to the saucepan, toasting it gently with the garlic for a minute or two. This step enhances the nutty flavor of the quinoa.

3. Pour in the vegetable or chicken broth, adding a pinch of salt and pepper. The broth will infuse the quinoa with savory goodness.

4. Bring the mixture to a boil, then reduce the heat to low. Cover the saucepan with a lid and let the quinoa simmer for about 15-20 minutes, or until the liquid is absorbed and the quinoa is tender.

5. Once cooked, remove the saucepan from the heat and let it sit, covered, for a few minutes. This allows the quinoa to fluff up and absorb any remaining moisture.

6. Fluff the quinoa with a fork, gently mixing in the chopped fresh herbs. The herbs will infuse the pilaf with a burst of freshness.

7. If desired, sprinkle in some lemon zest for an extra layer of brightness.

8. Serve the Fragrant Garlic and Herb Quinoa Pilaf in a dish, ready to be enjoyed.

9. For an added crunch, garnish with toasted nuts or seeds, adding both texture and a touch of nuttiness.

An Aromatic Symphony of Wholesome Goodness
Fragrant Garlic and Herb Quinoa Pilaf is more than just a dish; it's a symphony of aromas and flavors that showcases the beauty of simple, nourishing ingredients. With every forkful, you're not just enjoying a pilaf; you're savoring the subtle nuttiness of quinoa mingling with the rich warmth of garlic and the aromatic allure of fresh herbs.

This dish is a reminder that healthy meals can be both satisfying and full of character. By combining the nourishing power of quinoa with the aromatic embrace of garlic and herbs, you're creating a pilaf that's as pleasing to the palate as it is to your well-being.

So, whether you're relishing Fragrant Garlic and Herb Quinoa Pilaf as a wholesome side, using it as a base for vibrant bowls, or simply reveling in the joy of crafting a dish that tantalizes the senses and nourishes the body, let it be a reminder that the true art of cooking lies in the ability to create a symphony of flavors that resonate with both the palate and the soul.

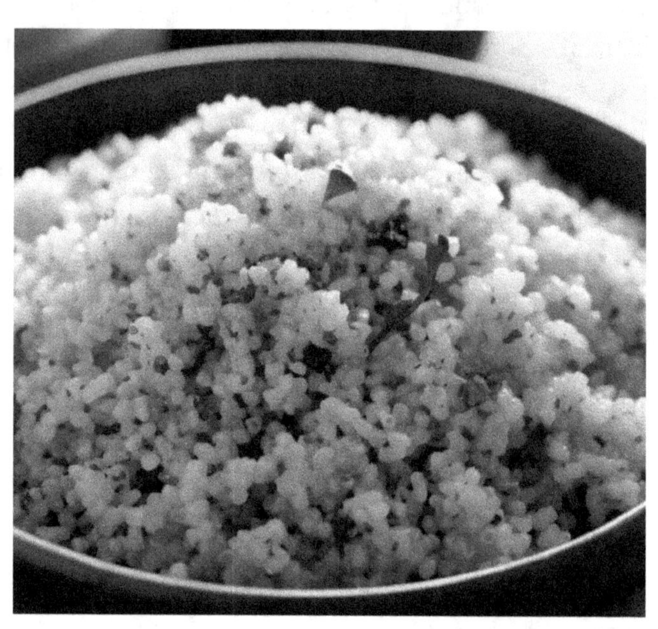

Spinach and Strawberry Salad with Tangy Balsamic Vinaigrette

Prepare to be delighted by a salad that captures the essence of the seasons and pairs it with a tantalizing burst of flavor. Our recipe for Spinach and Strawberry Salad with Tangy Balsamic Vinaigrette is a celebration of contrasts – the vibrant sweetness of strawberries mingling with the earthy notes of spinach, all united by a zesty balsamic vinaigrette. Get ready to embark on a culinary journey that's as refreshing as it is delectable.

Ingredients:
For the Spinach and Strawberry Salad:
- Fresh baby spinach leaves
- Ripe strawberries, hulled and sliced
- Red onion, thinly sliced
- Toasted nuts (such as almonds or walnuts), chopped
- Feta cheese or goat cheese, crumbled (optional)

For the Tangy Balsamic Vinaigrette:
- Balsamic vinegar
- Olive oil
- Dijon mustard
- Honey or maple syrup
- Garlic, minced
- Salt and pepper

Instructions:

For the Tangy Balsamic Vinaigrette:

1. In a small bowl, whisk together balsamic vinegar, Dijon mustard, honey or maple syrup, minced garlic, salt, and pepper. This harmonious blend will become the tangy dressing that brings the salad to life.

2. Slowly drizzle in the olive oil while whisking vigorously, creating a smooth and well-emulsified vinaigrette. The olive oil will add a luscious richness to the dressing.

3. Taste the vinaigrette and adjust the flavors to your liking, adding more honey for sweetness or more vinegar for tanginess.

For the Spinach and Strawberry Salad:

1. In a large salad bowl, place the fresh baby spinach leaves. Their vibrant green color sets the stage for the salad's visual appeal.

2. Scatter the sliced strawberries over the spinach, letting their natural sweetness add a burst of freshness.

3. Sprinkle the thinly sliced red onion and toasted nuts over the salad, adding layers of crunch and texture.

4. If using, crumble the feta cheese or goat cheese over the salad for a creamy contrast.

Bringing It All Together:
1. Give the Tangy Balsamic Vinaigrette a final whisk and drizzle it over the Spinach and Strawberry Salad.

2. Gently toss the salad to coat the ingredients with the flavorful dressing, ensuring every bite is kissed by the tangy vinaigrette.

3. As you take your first forkful, experience the symphony of flavors – the sweetness of strawberries dancing with the earthiness of spinach, all harmonized by the zesty vinaigrette.

A Medley of Taste and Texture
Spinach and Strawberry Salad with Tangy Balsamic Vinaigrette is more than just a salad; it's a medley of taste and texture that celebrates the art of balancing flavors. With every bite, you're not just consuming a dish; you're relishing a harmony that awakens your palate.

This salad is a reminder that simplicity can lead to extraordinary results. By pairing seasonal ingredients with a well-crafted vinaigrette, you're creating a salad that's not only a treat for your taste buds but also a celebration of freshness and balance.

So, whether you're savoring Spinach and Strawberry Salad with Tangy Balsamic Vinaigrette as a light and refreshing meal, sharing it with loved ones, or simply embracing the joy of crafting a dish that marries the best of nature's offerings, let it remind you that the true joy of cooking lies in the ability to transform ingredients into a symphony of flavors that sings on your palate and enriches your dining experience.

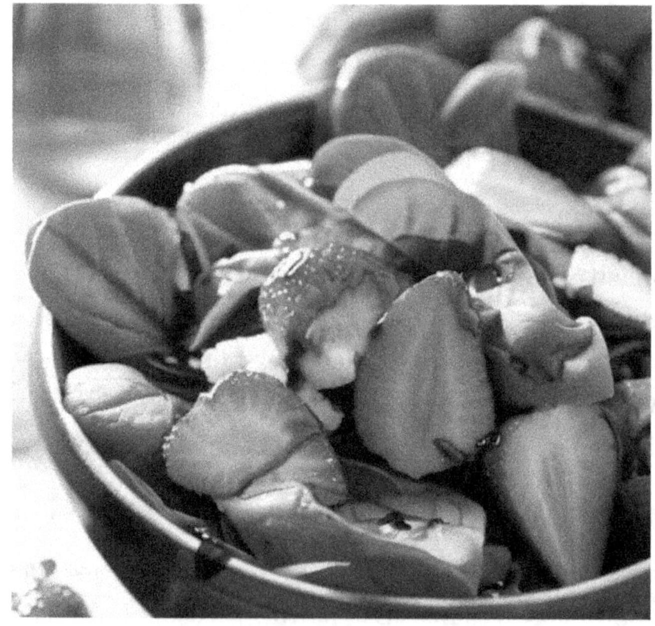

Chapter 8

Tasty Treats

Mini Banana Chocolate Chip Muffins for Little Hands

Indulge in a bite-sized delight that's perfect for both young and young-at-heart. Our recipe for Mini Banana Chocolate Chip Muffins brings together the timeless sweetness of ripe bananas and the irresistible allure of chocolate chips in a treat that's sure to bring smiles. Get ready to experience the joy of baking and the delight of enjoying these mini muffins that are just the right size for little hands.

Ingredients:
- Ripe bananas, mashed
- Flour (all-purpose or whole wheat)
- Baking powder
- Baking soda
- Salt
- Ground cinnamon
- Egg
- Brown sugar
- Milk (dairy or plant-based)

- Vanilla extract
- Chocolate chips

Instructions:

1. Preheat your oven to 350°F (175°C). Line a mini muffin tin with paper liners for easy removal.

2. In a bowl, whisk together the flour, baking powder, baking soda, salt, and ground cinnamon. This dry mixture will provide the structure and flavor of the muffins.

3. In a separate bowl, beat the egg and brown sugar together until well combined and slightly fluffy.

4. Add the mashed ripe bananas, milk, and vanilla extract to the egg and sugar mixture. Mix until everything is smoothly incorporated.

5. Gradually add the dry mixture to the wet mixture, gently folding until just combined. Be careful not to overmix, as this can make the muffins dense.

6. Gently fold in the chocolate chips, distributing them evenly throughout the batter for pockets of chocolatey goodness.

7. Using a mini ice cream scoop or two spoons, portion the muffin batter into the paper-lined muffin tin, filling each cup about two-thirds full.

8. Bake the mini muffins in the preheated oven for about 10-12 minutes, or until a toothpick inserted into the center comes out clean.

9. Once baked to perfection, remove the muffins from the oven and let them cool in the muffin tin for a few minutes before transferring them to a wire rack to cool completely.

A Bite-Sized Delight for All Ages
Mini Banana Chocolate Chip Muffins are more than just treats; they're a testament to the joy of baking and the pleasure of enjoying homemade goodness. With each tiny muffin, you're not just savoring a snack; you're indulging in a harmonious blend of comforting bananas and the allure of chocolate.

This recipe is a reminder that even the smallest treats can create the biggest smiles. By crafting mini muffins that are perfectly sized for little hands, you're creating an experience that's not only delicious but also tailored to the delight of young ones.

So, whether you're sharing Mini Banana Chocolate Chip Muffins as an after-school treat, packing them for on-the-go munching, or simply embracing the art of baking with love, let them be a reminder that the simple pleasures of life are often the ones that bring the greatest joy.

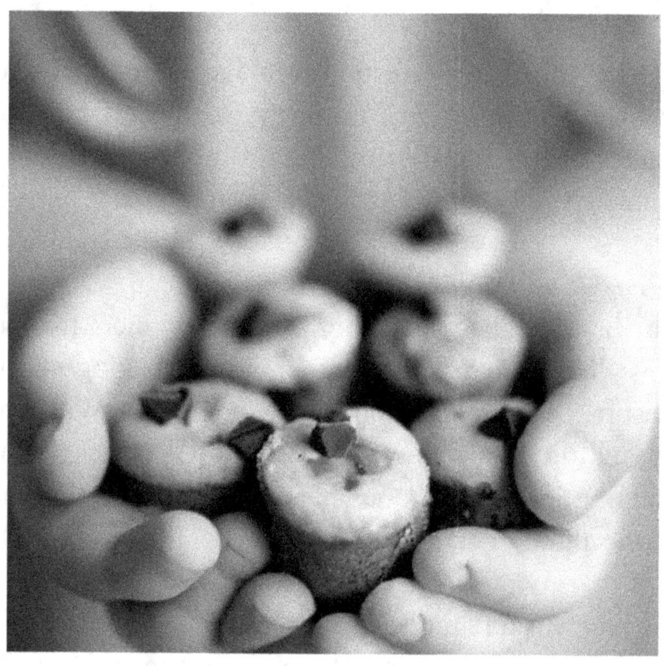

Berry Blast Frozen Yogurt Pops for Cooling Delight

Quench your cravings with a frozen delight that's as vibrant in taste as it is in color. Our recipe for Berry Blast Frozen Yogurt Pops brings you the essence of summer's bounty, transforming a medley of berries into a frozen treat that's both cooling and invigorating. Get ready to experience a burst of fruity joy that will have you embracing the sweet pleasures of the season.

Ingredients:
- Mixed berries (strawberries, blueberries, raspberries, blackberries), fresh or frozen
- Greek yogurt or your choice of yogurt
- Honey or maple syrup, for sweetness (optional)
- Lemon juice (optional)

Instructions:
1. In a blender, combine the mixed berries. If using frozen berries, allow them to thaw slightly before blending.

2. Blend the berries until they're smooth and pureed, creating a vibrant berry sauce that's bursting with natural sweetness.

3. If desired, add a touch of honey or maple syrup to the berry puree, enhancing its sweetness. A squeeze of lemon juice can also be added to balance the flavors and add a zesty twist.

4. In a separate bowl, mix the berry puree with Greek yogurt or your choice of yogurt. The combination of yogurt and berry puree will create a swirl of color and flavor.

5. Taste the mixture and adjust the sweetness level if needed, keeping in mind that freezing will slightly dull the sweetness.

6. Carefully pour the berry and yogurt mixture into popsicle molds, allowing room for expansion as they freeze.

7. Insert popsicle sticks into the molds and place them in the freezer. Allow the pops to freeze for several hours or until they're solid.

8. Once frozen, remove the Berry Blast Frozen Yogurt Pops from the molds by running them briefly under warm water to release the popsicles.

A Symphony of Coolness and Flavor

Berry Blast Frozen Yogurt Pops are more than just a frozen treat; they're a symphony of coolness and flavor that encapsulates the joy of summer. With each lick, you're not just enjoying a popsicle; you're savoring the natural sweetness of berries in a refreshing and delightful form.

This recipe is a reminder that indulgence can be both nourishing and satisfying. By using wholesome ingredients like mixed berries and yogurt, and by controlling the level of sweetness, you're creating a frozen delight that's kind to your taste buds and your well-being.

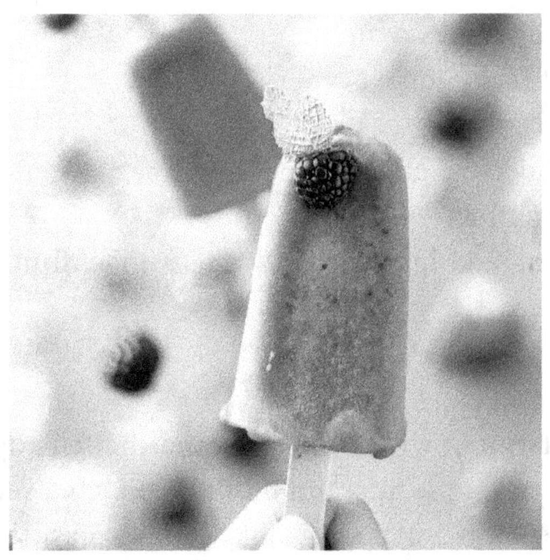

Nut Butter Energy Bites for Sustained Energy

Elevate your snacking game with a treat that's not only delectable but also fuels your body with a burst of sustained energy. Our recipe for Nut Butter Energy Bites is a celebration of natural ingredients that come together to create a bite-sized powerhouse of vitality. Get ready to experience a snack that's as delightful to your taste buds as it is nourishing for your well-being.

Ingredients:

- Nut butter of your choice (almond, peanut, cashew, etc.)
- Rolled oats
- Honey or maple syrup
- Ground flaxseed
- Chia seeds
- Dark chocolate chips or cocoa nibs
- Vanilla extract
- Optional add-ins: chopped nuts, dried fruit, coconut flakes

Instructions:

1. In a large bowl, combine the nut butter, rolled oats, honey or maple syrup, ground flaxseed, chia seeds, dark chocolate chips or cocoa nibs, and a splash of vanilla extract.

2. Mix the ingredients until they're well combined and form a cohesive mixture. The nut butter will provide the binding factor for the energy bites.

3. If you're including optional add-ins like chopped nuts, dried fruit, or coconut flakes, fold them into the mixture to add extra texture and flavor.

4. Once the mixture is ready, refrigerate it for about 30 minutes. This will make it easier to handle when shaping the energy bites.

5. After chilling, take spoonfuls of the mixture and roll them into bite-sized balls between your palms. You can adjust the size to your preference.

6. Place the formed Nut Butter Energy Bites on a baking sheet or plate lined with parchment paper.

7. Refrigerate the energy bites for an additional 30 minutes to allow them to set and firm up.

8. Once they're chilled and firm, transfer the Nut Butter Energy Bites to an airtight container for storage.

Nut Butter Energy Bites are more than just a snack; they're a testament to the power of whole foods in boosting your energy levels. With every bite, you're not just enjoying a treat; you're providing your body with a combination of nutrients that's designed to keep you fueled and focused.

This snack is a reminder that eating for energy doesn't mean sacrificing taste. By combining the richness of nut butter, the heartiness of oats, and the benefits of seeds, you're crafting a convenient and satisfying source of vitality.

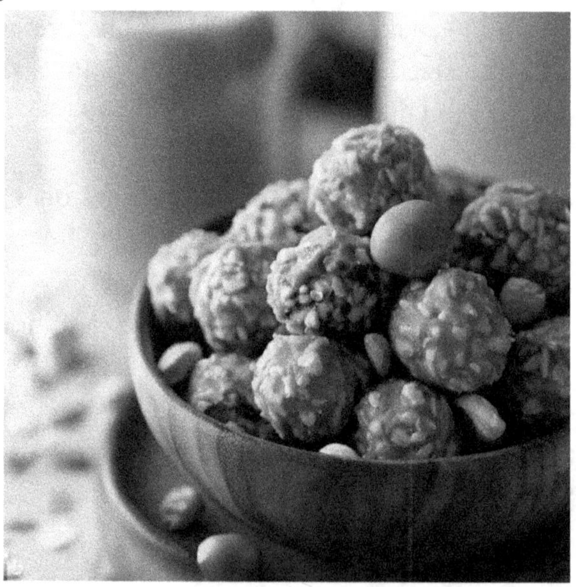

Chapter 9

Family-Friendly Desserts

Baked Apples with Cinnamon and Crunchy Walnuts

Indulge in the sweetness of a dessert that's not only delightful to the taste buds but also brings a touch of warmth and comfort to your family table. Our recipe for Baked Apples with Cinnamon and Crunchy Walnuts is a celebration of simplicity and heartwarming flavors that create a dessert as satisfying as it is wholesome. Prepare to savor a treat that's perfect for family gatherings, cozy evenings, and any occasion that calls for a touch of sweetness.

Ingredients:
- Apples (such as Granny Smith, Honeycrisp, or Fuji)
- Ground cinnamon
- Chopped walnuts
- Honey or maple syrup
- Optional add-ins: dried cranberries, raisins, chopped dates

Instructions:

1. Preheat your oven to 375°F (190°C).

2. Start by preparing the apples. Wash and core them, removing the center seeds and creating a cavity for the filling.

3. In a bowl, mix the chopped walnuts with a sprinkle of ground cinnamon. The cinnamon will infuse the walnuts with a cozy aroma.

4. If you're including optional add-ins like dried cranberries, raisins, or chopped dates, fold them into the walnut mixture to add a burst of sweetness and texture.

5. Fill the cavities of the cored apples with the cinnamon-infused walnut mixture, pressing it gently to create a snug fit.

6. Place the filled apples in a baking dish, ensuring they're stable and won't tip over.

7. Drizzle each apple with a touch of honey or maple syrup, letting the natural sweetness enhance the dessert.

8. Sprinkle a bit more ground cinnamon over the top of each apple for an extra layer of flavor.

9. Cover the baking dish with foil and bake the apples in the preheated oven for about 20-25 minutes, or until they're tender but still hold their shape.

10. Once baked to perfection, remove the apples from the oven and let them cool slightly before serving.

Bringing Comfort and Flavor to Your Table
Baked Apples with Cinnamon and Crunchy Walnuts are more than just a dessert; they're a gesture of warmth and love that graces your family gatherings. With every bite, you're not just enjoying a treat; you're savoring the nostalgia of baked goods, the comforting scent of cinnamon, and the delightful crunch of walnuts.

This dessert is a reminder that family-friendly treats can be both satisfying and nourishing. By using wholesome ingredients like apples and nuts, and infusing them with the richness of cinnamon, you're creating a dessert that's as heartwarming as it is delicious.

So, whether you're savoring Baked Apples with Cinnamon and Crunchy Walnuts as a heartwarming finish to a meal, sharing them with loved ones on cozy evenings, or simply relishing the joy of creating a dessert that embodies the essence of comfort and togetherness, let them remind you that the true essence of a family dessert lies in the ability to bring smiles, warmth, and the sweetness of shared moments to your table.

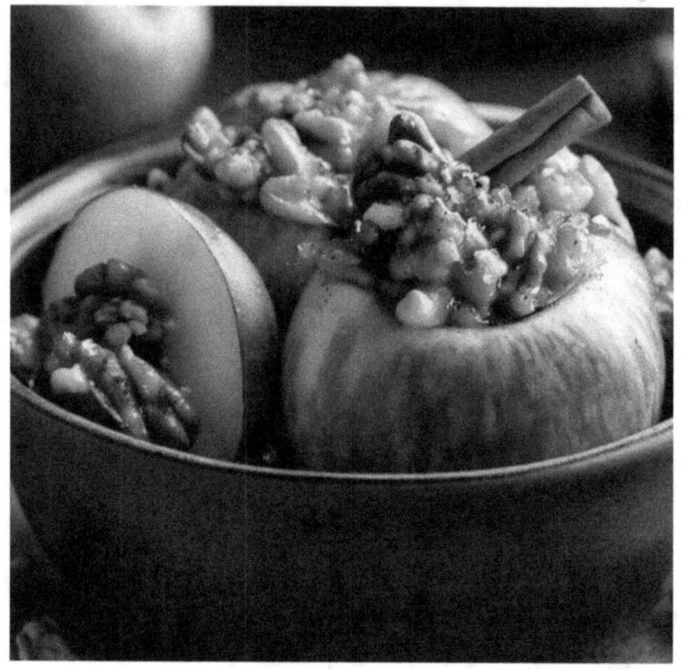

Mixed Berry Crumble with Wholesome Oat Topping

Indulge in the heartwarming embrace of a dessert that brings together the sweetness of mixed berries and the rustic charm of a wholesome oat topping. Our recipe for Mixed Berry Crumble is a celebration of flavors and textures that dance in harmony, creating a dessert that's as cozy as it is delicious. Get ready to experience a treat that captures the essence of comfort and indulgence.

Ingredients:
For the Mixed Berry Filling:
- Mixed berries (strawberries, blueberries, raspberries, blackberries), fresh or frozen
- Lemon zest and juice
- Honey or maple syrup
- Cornstarch or arrowroot powder

For the Wholesome Oat Topping:
- Rolled oats
- Whole wheat flour
- Chopped nuts (such as almonds, walnuts, or pecans)
- Coconut oil or butter
- Honey or maple syrup
- Ground cinnamon
- Pinch of salt

Instructions:

For the Mixed Berry Filling:

1. Preheat your oven to 375°F (190°C).

2. In a bowl, combine the mixed berries, lemon zest, lemon juice, and a drizzle of honey or maple syrup. These ingredients will create a vibrant and naturally sweet filling.

3. Sprinkle the cornstarch or arrowroot powder over the berries, tossing gently to coat them. This will help thicken the berry juices as they bake.

4. Transfer the berry mixture to a baking dish, spreading it evenly to create a luscious base for the crumble topping.

For the Wholesome Oat Topping:

1. In a bowl, combine the rolled oats, whole wheat flour, chopped nuts, ground cinnamon, and a pinch of salt. The oats and nuts will provide a delightful crunch to the topping.

2. In a small saucepan, melt the coconut oil or butter over low heat. Once melted, add a drizzle of honey or maple syrup, stirring to combine.

3. Pour the coconut oil mixture over the dry oat mixture and mix until everything is well coated. The mixture should resemble coarse crumbs.

Assembling the Crumble:
1. Evenly spread the Wholesome Oat Topping over the Mixed Berry Filling, covering it with a generous layer of the oat mixture.

2. Place the baking dish in the preheated oven and bake for about 25-30 minutes, or until the berry filling is bubbling and the oat topping is golden and crisp.

3. Once baked to perfection, remove the Mixed Berry Crumble from the oven and let it cool slightly before serving.

A Heartwarming Fusion of Flavors
Mixed Berry Crumble with Wholesome Oat Topping is more than just a dessert; it's a fusion of flavors that evokes the comfort of home-cooked goodness. With every spoonful, you're not just savoring a treat; you're experiencing the sweetness of mixed berries melding with the warmth of cinnamon-spiced oats.

This dessert is a reminder that indulgence can be both comforting and nourishing. By using a medley of mixed berries and creating a rustic oat topping, you're crafting a dessert that's as wholesome as it is satisfying.

So, whether you're savoring Mixed Berry Crumble as a heartwarming dessert, sharing it with loved ones on special occasions, or simply embracing the joy of baking with the flavors of the season, let it remind you that the magic of a dessert lies in the ability to infuse every bite with love, comfort, and the sweet delight of shared moments.

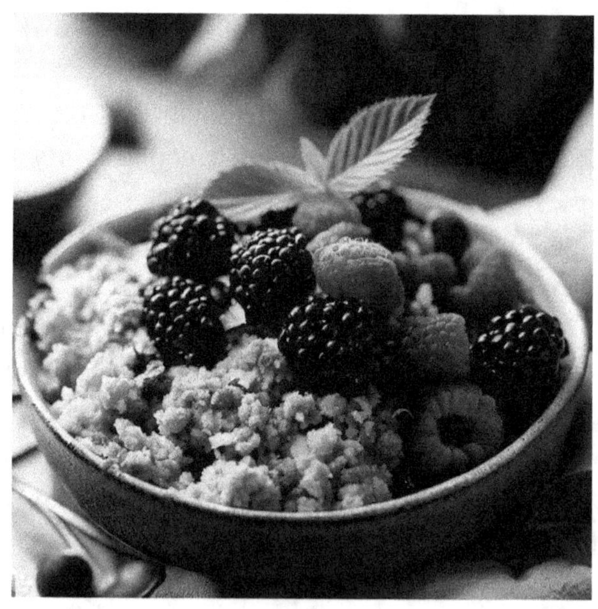

Chocolate-Dipped Fruit Kabobs for Festive Occasions

Elevate your festivities with a treat that's not only visually appealing but also irresistibly delicious. Our recipe for Chocolate-Dipped Fruit Kabobs brings together the vibrant colors of fresh fruits and the decadence of chocolate, creating a dessert that's perfect for special occasions and celebrations. Prepare to savor a delightful combination of flavors and textures that's sure to add a touch of elegance and joy to any gathering.

Ingredients:
- Assorted fresh fruits (strawberries, bananas, pineapple, kiwi, etc.), cut into bite-sized pieces
- Dark chocolate or milk chocolate, melted
- Wooden skewers

Instructions:
1. Prepare the fresh fruits by washing, peeling, and cutting them into bite-sized pieces. The assortment of colors and flavors will create a visually stunning display.

2. Line a baking sheet with parchment paper to place the prepared fruit kabobs on.

3. Melt the chocolate using a double boiler or in short bursts in the microwave. Stir until smooth and creamy.

4. Carefully thread the fruit pieces onto the wooden skewers, alternating colors and varieties to create an attractive pattern.

5. Dip each fruit skewer into the melted chocolate, ensuring that the fruit is coated about halfway. You can dip them fully for a more indulgent treat if desired.

6. Allow any excess chocolate to drip off before placing the dipped fruit kabobs on the prepared baking sheet.

7. If you'd like to add an extra touch of decoration, you can drizzle a bit more melted chocolate over the dipped fruit or sprinkle with chopped nuts or coconut flakes.

8. Place the baking sheet in the refrigerator for about 20-30 minutes, or until the chocolate is set and the fruit is secure on the skewers.

Bringing Elegance and Flavor to Your Table
Chocolate-Dipped Fruit Kabobs are more than just a dessert; they're a celebration of taste and aesthetics that adds a touch of elegance to your festive occasions. With every bite, you're not just enjoying a treat; you're savoring the harmonious contrast of luscious fruits and rich chocolate.

This dessert is a reminder that indulgence can be both beautiful and delectable. By combining the goodness of fresh fruits with the velvety allure of melted chocolate, you're creating a dessert that's sure to captivate the senses of your guests.

So, whether you're serving Chocolate-Dipped Fruit Kabobs as a stunning dessert centerpiece at a gathering, using them to add a touch of sophistication to a party, or simply embracing the joy of creating edible works of art, let them remind you that celebrations are made sweeter when paired with the magic of flavor and the art of presentation.

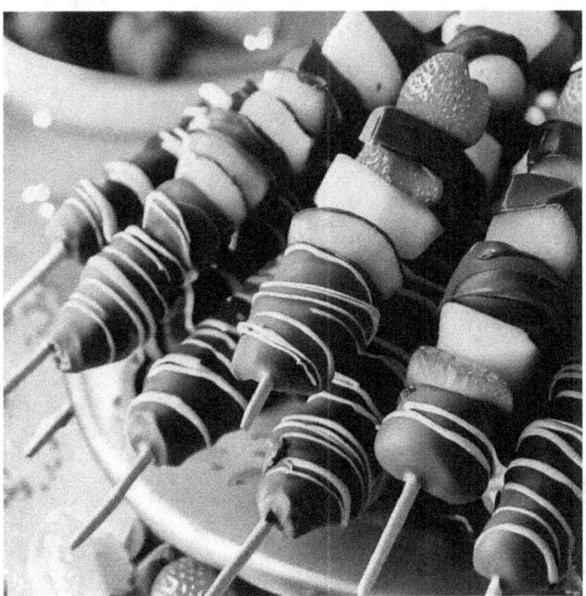

Creamy Chocolate Avocado Pudding for Guilt-Free Indulgence

Satisfy your chocolate cravings without compromise as you dive into a dessert that's as creamy as it is guilt-free. Our recipe for Creamy Chocolate Avocado Pudding is a celebration of rich flavors and wholesome ingredients that come together to create a luscious treat that's perfect for indulging in without hesitation. Prepare to experience a dessert that's as delightful to your taste buds as it is kind to your well-being.

Ingredients:
- Ripe avocados, peeled and pitted
- Cocoa powder (unsweetened)
- Honey or maple syrup
- Vanilla extract
- A pinch of salt
- Optional add-ins: almond milk, banana, nut butter, chia seeds

Instructions:

1. In a food processor or blender, combine the ripe avocados, unsweetened cocoa powder, a drizzle of honey or maple syrup, a splash of vanilla extract, and a pinch of salt.

2. Blend the ingredients until they're smooth and creamy, forming a decadent chocolate mixture. The natural creaminess of avocados will lend a velvety texture to the pudding.

3. Taste the pudding and adjust the sweetness to your preference by adding more honey or maple syrup if desired.

4. If you're opting for optional add-ins like almond milk for extra creaminess, a banana for natural sweetness, nut butter for richness, or chia seeds for added texture, blend them into the mixture until well incorporated.

5. Once the pudding is smooth and well combined, transfer it to serving dishes or individual cups.

6. Refrigerate the pudding for about an hour to allow it to chill and set, enhancing its creamy consistency.

7. Before serving, you can garnish the Creamy Chocolate Avocado Pudding with a sprinkle of cocoa powder, grated chocolate, fresh berries, or a dollop of whipped cream for an extra touch of indulgence.

Indulgence without the Guilt
Creamy Chocolate Avocado Pudding is more than just a dessert; it's a testament to how indulgence and health can

beautifully coexist. With every spoonful, you're not just relishing a treat; you're embracing the rich flavors of chocolate and the creamy goodness of avocados in a guilt-free package.

This dessert is a reminder that you don't have to compromise on taste to make a healthful choice. By harnessing the nutritional power of avocados and the joy of chocolate, you're creating a dessert that's as satisfying to your palate as it is kind to your body.

So, whether you're savoring Creamy Chocolate Avocado Pudding as a delectable end to a meal, sharing it with loved ones, or simply enjoying the pleasure of a dessert that's both indulgent and nourishing, let it be your reminder that the delight of eating can be as enriching as it is delightful – a truly indulgent experience that nurtures both your cravings and your well-being.

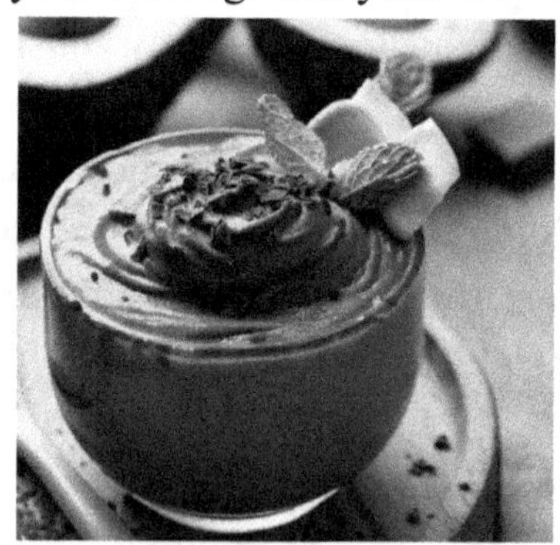

Chapter 10

Drinks and Beverages

Refreshing Watermelon Limeade for Hydration

Experience the ultimate refresher that not only quenches your thirst but also invigorates your senses with the pure essence of summer. Our recipe for Refreshing Watermelon Limeade is a celebration of hydration and natural flavors that come together to create a revitalizing drink that's as delicious as it is replenishing. Get ready to sip on a beverage that's perfect for sunny days, outdoor gatherings, or any moment when you seek a burst of rejuvenation.

Ingredients:

- Fresh watermelon, cubed and seeds removed
- Freshly squeezed lime juice
- Honey or agave syrup
- Fresh mint leaves
- Ice cubes
- Sparkling water or still water

Instructions:

1. In a blender, combine the fresh watermelon cubes and a splash of freshly squeezed lime juice.

2. Blend the watermelon until it's smooth and liquid, forming a vibrant and hydrating base for your limeade.

3. Taste the watermelon mixture and add a drizzle of honey or agave syrup if you'd like a touch of sweetness. This step is adjustable based on your preference for sweetness.

4. For an extra burst of freshness, tear a few fresh mint leaves and add them to the blender. Blend briefly to infuse the minty aroma into the mixture.

5. Strain the watermelon mixture through a fine mesh strainer to remove any remaining pulp or seeds, if desired.

6. Fill glasses with ice cubes to keep your limeade wonderfully chilled.

7. Pour the strained watermelon mixture over the ice, filling each glass about halfway.

8. Top off the glasses with either sparkling water or still water, adjusting the amount based on your desired level of fizziness.

9. Garnish the Refreshing Watermelon Limeade with a slice of lime and a sprig of fresh mint for a touch of elegance.

Hydration with a Twist of Flavor

Refreshing Watermelon Limeade is more than just a drink; it's a celebration of the natural bounty of summer that's designed to hydrate and delight. With every sip, you're not just quenching your thirst; you're immersing yourself in the juicy sweetness of watermelon and the tangy zing of lime.

This limeade is a reminder that hydration can be both a necessity and an indulgence. By harnessing the juicy goodness of watermelon and the invigorating tang of lime, you're creating a beverage that's as rejuvenating as it is enjoyable.

So, whether you're sipping Refreshing Watermelon Limeade as a revitalizing pick-me-up, sharing it with friends and family during gatherings, or simply embracing the joy of a beverage that refreshes both your body and your spirit, let it be your reminder that the simple act of staying hydrated can be a flavorful journey of quenching, sipping, and savoring the essence of summer.

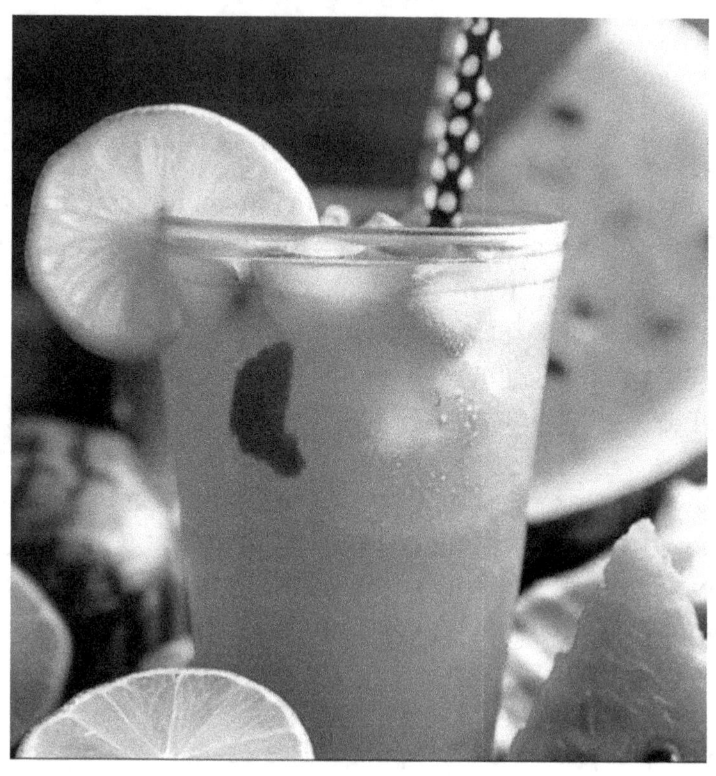

Bursting Berry Blast Smoothie for Nutrient Boost

Elevate your mornings and recharge your day with a smoothie that's as vibrant as it is nourishing. Our recipe for Bursting Berry Blast Smoothie is a celebration of the bold flavors and wholesome goodness that berries bring to your glass. Get ready to experience a blend that's not only a treat for your taste buds but also a powerhouse of nutrients that fuel your body with vitality.

Ingredients:
- Mixed berries (strawberries, blueberries, raspberries, blackberries)
- Banana
- Greek yogurt or dairy-free yogurt
- Almond milk or your preferred milk
- Honey or maple syrup
- Ground flaxseed or chia seeds (optional)
- Ice cubes

Instructions:
1. Start by adding a handful of mixed berries to the blender. The combination of different berries brings a symphony of flavors and a burst of antioxidants.

2. Peel and slice a ripe banana, adding it to the blender. The banana not only adds natural sweetness but also contributes to the creamy texture of the smoothie.

3. Spoon in a generous portion of Greek yogurt or dairy-free yogurt. The yogurt adds creaminess and a dose of probiotics.

4. Pour in almond milk or your preferred milk to achieve your desired level of thickness. The milk will help create a smooth consistency for your smoothie.

5. Drizzle a touch of honey or maple syrup for added sweetness, if desired. Adjust the amount based on your preference.

6. If you're looking to boost the nutrition, add ground flaxseed or chia seeds to the blender. These seeds are rich in fiber and healthy fats.

7. Add a handful of ice cubes to the blender to create a refreshingly chilled and invigorating smoothie.

8. Blend the ingredients on high speed until they're well combined and the smoothie is smooth and velvety.

9. Taste the smoothie and adjust the sweetness by adding more honey or maple syrup if needed.

10. Pour the Bursting Berry Blast Smoothie into glasses, ready to be enjoyed.

Flavorful Nutrient Powerhouse
Bursting Berry Blast Smoothie is more than just a drink; it's a nutritional powerhouse that's designed to awaken your taste buds and provide your body with a burst of nourishment. With every sip, you're not just savoring the delightful medley of berries; you're also benefiting from their vitamins, minerals, and antioxidants.

This smoothie is a reminder that nourishing your body can be as delicious as it is essential. By blending together a variety of berries, creamy yogurt, and other nutritious ingredients, you're creating a beverage that's both satisfying and revitalizing.

So, whether you're enjoying Bursting Berry Blast Smoothie as a wholesome breakfast, refueling after a workout, or simply embracing the joy of a drink that energizes your body and delights your palate, let it be your reminder that nutrient-rich choices can be both delicious and invigorating – a true whirlwind of flavor and nourishment in every sip.

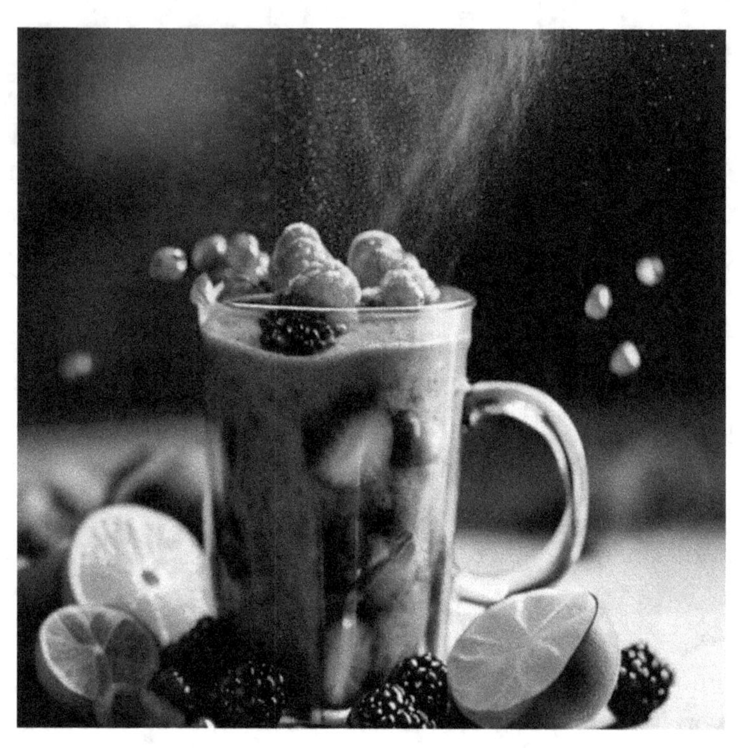

Chapter 11

Special Occasion Treats

Whole Wheat Veggie Pizza for Flavorful Celebrations

Elevate your special moments with a dish that's not only delicious but also a reflection of wholesome indulgence. Our recipe for Whole Wheat Veggie Pizza is a celebration of flavors and the joy of sharing a meal with loved ones. Get ready to savor a pizza that's not only a feast for your taste buds but also a delightful centerpiece for any occasion worth celebrating.

Ingredients:
For the Whole Wheat Pizza Dough:
- Whole wheat flour
- Active dry yeast
- Warm water
- Olive oil
- Honey or maple syrup
- Salt

For the Veggie Pizza Toppings:
- Tomato sauce or pesto sauce

- A colorful variety of vegetables (bell peppers, cherry tomatoes, red onion, zucchini, etc.)
- Mozzarella cheese or your favorite cheese
- Fresh basil leaves
- Olive oil
- Dried oregano
- Salt and pepper

Instructions:

For the Whole Wheat Pizza Dough:

1. In a bowl, dissolve the active dry yeast in warm water and let it sit for a few minutes until it's frothy.

2. Add honey or maple syrup, olive oil, and a pinch of salt to the yeast mixture. Mix well to combine.

3. Gradually add whole wheat flour, stirring until the dough comes together.

4. Turn the dough onto a floured surface and knead it for a few minutes until it's smooth and elastic.

5. Place the dough in a greased bowl, cover it with a damp cloth, and let it rise in a warm place until it doubles in size.

For the Veggie Pizza:

1. Preheat your oven to the temperature recommended for pizza baking (usually around 450°F or 230°C).

2. Roll out the risen whole wheat pizza dough on a floured surface to your desired thickness and shape.

3. Transfer the rolled-out dough to a baking sheet or pizza stone.

4. Spread a layer of tomato sauce or pesto sauce over the dough, leaving a border around the edges for the crust.

5. Arrange a colorful variety of sliced vegetables over the sauce.

6. Sprinkle grated mozzarella cheese or your preferred cheese over the vegetables.

7. Drizzle a bit of olive oil over the toppings and sprinkle dried oregano, salt, and pepper for extra flavor.

8. Slide the prepared pizza into the preheated oven and bake it until the crust is golden and the cheese is bubbly and melted.

9. Once baked, remove the pizza from the oven and let it cool slightly before slicing.

10. Before serving, scatter fresh basil leaves over the pizza for a fragrant and vibrant finish.

Celebrating with Flavor and Wholesomeness
Whole Wheat Veggie Pizza is more than just a dish; it's a celebration of taste, togetherness, and the art of creating memories around the table. With every bite, you're not just enjoying a pizza; you're relishing the harmony of whole wheat crust, vibrant vegetables, melted cheese, and the aroma of fresh basil.

This pizza is a reminder that special occasions deserve food that's both satisfying and nourishing. By crafting a pizza that showcases whole wheat goodness and the freshness of colorful vegetables, you're creating a centerpiece that's as heartwarming as it is delectable.

So, whether you're sharing Whole Wheat Veggie Pizza at festive gatherings, using it to mark cherished moments, or simply embracing the joy of a dish that captures the essence of celebration, let it be a reminder that every occasion is made even more special with food that brings people together and fills the air with the aroma of love and deliciousness.

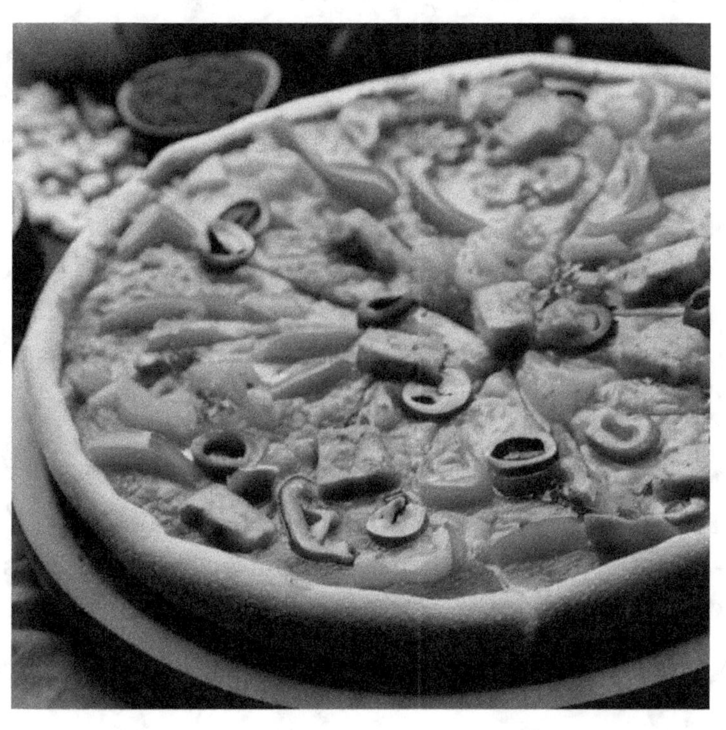

Baked Chicken Tenders with Zesty Honey Mustard Dip

Elevate your comfort food game with a dish that combines the satisfaction of crispy chicken tenders with the zing of a zesty honey mustard dip. Our recipe for Baked Chicken Tenders with Zesty Honey Mustard Dip is a celebration of flavors and textures that come together to create a meal that's both satisfying and irresistibly delicious. Get ready to indulge in a dish that's perfect for family dinners, game nights, or any occasion that calls for finger-licking goodness.

Ingredients:
For the Baked Chicken Tenders:
- Chicken tenders or boneless, skinless chicken breasts, cut into strips
- Bread crumbs (regular or panko)
- Parmesan cheese, grated (optional)
- Garlic powder
- Paprika
- Salt and pepper
- Eggs, beaten

For the Zesty Honey Mustard Dip:
- Dijon mustard
- Honey
- Lemon juice

- Mayonnaise or Greek yogurt
- Salt and pepper

Instructions:
For the Baked Chicken Tenders:
1. Preheat your oven to 400°F (200°C). Line a baking sheet with parchment paper to prevent sticking.

2. In a bowl, combine the bread crumbs, grated Parmesan cheese (if using), garlic powder, paprika, salt, and pepper. This mixture will create a flavorful coating for your chicken tenders.

3. Dip each chicken tender into the beaten eggs, allowing any excess to drip off.

4. Roll the egg-coated chicken tender in the breadcrumb mixture, pressing gently to ensure the coating adheres.

5. Place the coated chicken tenders on the prepared baking sheet, ensuring they're spaced apart for even baking.

6. Bake the chicken tenders in the preheated oven for about 15-20 minutes, flipping them halfway through, until they're golden and cooked through.

For the Zesty Honey Mustard Dip:

1. In a bowl, whisk together Dijon mustard, honey, lemon juice, mayonnaise or Greek yogurt, salt, and pepper. The combination of tangy Dijon and the sweetness of honey creates a balanced and flavorful dip.

2. Taste the dip and adjust the seasonings to your preference, adding more honey or mustard if desired.

3. Refrigerate the dip until you're ready to serve.

Bringing Flavorful Comfort to the Table

Baked Chicken Tenders with Zesty Honey Mustard Dip is more than just a meal; it's a symphony of textures and flavors that cater to both your comfort cravings and your taste for tangy delight. With every bite, you're not just savoring the crispy exterior of the chicken; you're also dipping into the zesty notes of honey mustard.

This dish is a reminder that comfort food can be both satisfying and enjoyable. By baking instead of deep-frying the chicken tenders and by creating a zesty dip with a perfect balance of flavors, you're crafting a meal that's as delicious as it is nourishing.

So, whether you're enjoying Baked Chicken Tenders with Zesty Honey Mustard Dip as a delightful main course, sharing it with loved ones during gatherings, or simply embracing the joy of a meal that brings smiles and finger-licking satisfaction, let it be your reminder that comfort and flavor can coexist in a dish that's both irresistible and comforting.

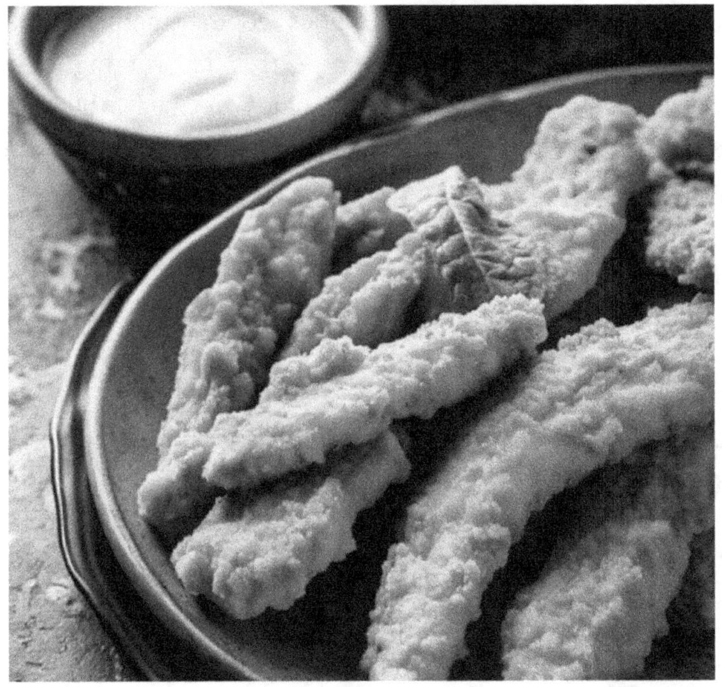

Veggie and Cheese Quesadillas for Flavorful Gatherings

Gather around the table and experience the joy of sharing a dish that's both flavorful and comforting. Our recipe for Veggie and Cheese Quesadillas is a celebration of vibrant ingredients and ooey-gooey goodness that come together to create a dish perfect for bringing loved ones together. Get ready to enjoy a meal that's as satisfying to the taste buds as it is heartwarming for the soul.

Ingredients:
- Flour tortillas (medium-sized)
- Mixed vegetables (bell peppers, onions, zucchini, mushrooms, etc.), sliced
- Shredded cheese (cheddar, Monterey Jack, or your favorite melting cheese)
- Olive oil
- Mexican seasoning blend (cumin, chili powder, paprika, etc.)
- Salt and pepper
- Optional add-ins: black beans, corn, jalapenos, avocado slices

Instructions:
1. In a skillet over medium heat, add a drizzle of olive oil. Sauté the sliced mixed vegetables until they're tender

and slightly caramelized. Sprinkle the Mexican seasoning blend, salt, and pepper over the veggies to infuse them with bold flavors.

2. Once the veggies are cooked to perfection, transfer them to a plate and set them aside.

3. In the same skillet, lay down a flour tortilla. Sprinkle a layer of shredded cheese evenly over half of the tortilla.

4. Spread a generous portion of the sautéed vegetables over the cheese.

5. Sprinkle another layer of shredded cheese over the veggies, creating a gooey sandwich between the tortilla halves.

6. Fold the tortilla in half, covering the cheesy and veggie-filled side.

7. Cook the quesadilla in the skillet for a few minutes on each side, until the tortilla is golden and crispy, and the cheese is melted to perfection.

8. Remove the quesadilla from the skillet and let it rest for a moment before slicing it into wedges.

9. Repeat the process for the remaining tortillas, veggies, and cheese.

Flavorful Comfort for Gatherings
Veggie and Cheese Quesadillas are more than just a dish; they're a representation of togetherness and shared delight that graces your gatherings. With every bite, you're not just savoring the melty goodness of cheese and the burst of flavors from the veggies; you're also experiencing the joy of coming together around a delicious meal.

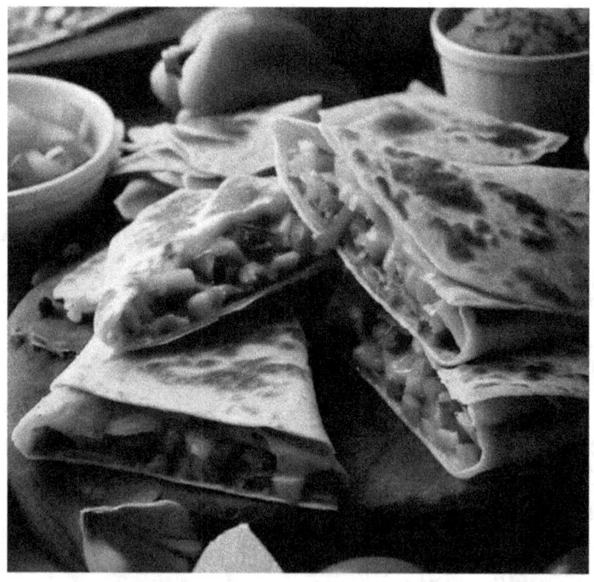

Chapter 12

Tips for Managing Blood Sugar

Mastering Portion Control and Smart Carb Counting

Embarking on a journey to manage your blood sugar doesn't mean giving up on the joy of eating. Instead, it's an opportunity to learn how to make mindful choices that can lead to better health and well-being. In this section, we'll delve into two essential aspects of managing blood sugar – mastering portion control and adopting smart carb counting techniques. By understanding these principles, you'll be empowered to make informed decisions that positively impact your blood sugar levels while still savoring the pleasures of food.

Portion control is about understanding the right amount of food to consume, ensuring that you strike a balance between enjoying your meals and maintaining stable blood sugar levels. Here's how you can master portion control:

1. Listen to Your Body: Pay attention to hunger and fullness cues. Eat slowly and savor each bite, giving your body time to signal when it's satisfied.

2. Use Smaller Plates and Bowls: Opt for smaller plates and bowls to create the illusion of a fuller plate. This can help you feel satisfied with smaller portions.

3. Plate Mindfully: Fill half of your plate with non-starchy vegetables, a quarter with lean protein, and a quarter with complex carbohydrates.

4. Avoid Eating Directly from Containers: Portion out your food onto a plate to prevent overeating. This practice also allows you to appreciate the visual appeal of your meal.

5. Check In with Hunger Levels: Before reaching for seconds, assess whether you're truly hungry or if you're eating out of habit or boredom.

Smart Carb Counting: Making Informed Choices
Carbohydrates have a direct impact on blood sugar levels. However, not all carbs are created equal. Smart carb counting involves choosing carbohydrates that have a gentler effect on blood sugar. Here's how you can make informed carb choices:

1. Choose Whole Grains: Opt for whole grains like brown rice, quinoa, whole wheat pasta, and whole grain bread. These contain fiber that slows down digestion and stabilizes blood sugar.

2. Favor Low Glycemic Index Foods: Foods with a low glycemic index (GI) release glucose slowly, preventing rapid spikes in blood sugar. Examples include legumes, non-starchy vegetables, and most fruits.

3. Pair Carbs with Protein and Healthy Fats: Combining carbohydrates with protein and healthy fats can help mitigate their impact on blood sugar. For instance, have an apple with almond butter for a balanced snack.

4. Read Nutrition Labels: Pay attention to total carbohydrates and serving sizes on nutrition labels. This information is key to managing carb intake.

5. Monitor Blood Sugar Responses: Over time, observe how different foods affect your blood sugar levels. This personalized knowledge can guide your food choices.

Empowering Yourself for Long-Term Success
Mastering portion control and adopting smart carb counting techniques empowers you to take charge of

your blood sugar management journey. By focusing on quality over quantity and making mindful carb choices, you're making strides toward improved well-being without sacrificing the enjoyment of food. Remember, every meal is an opportunity to nourish your body and make choices that align with your health goals. As you incorporate these principles into your eating habits, you'll find that managing blood sugar becomes a seamless part of your lifestyle, allowing you to savor life's flavors while prioritizing your health.

Swapping Ingredients for a Healthier Culinary Journey

Embarking on a journey towards healthier eating doesn't mean saying goodbye to your favorite dishes. It's about discovering creative ways to swap ingredients without compromising on taste and enjoyment. In this section, we'll explore the art of ingredient substitution, empowering you to transform your culinary creations into nourishing delights that support your well-being.

Swapping ingredients is an exciting opportunity to infuse your meals with greater nutritional value. By making thoughtful choices, you can reduce saturated fats, sugar, and refined carbohydrates, while increasing fiber, vitamins, and minerals. The key is to find alternatives that maintain the essence of your dish while enhancing its healthfulness.

Simple Ingredient Swaps for Everyday Cooking
1. Whole Grains for Refined Grains: Replace white rice, pasta, and bread with their whole grain counterparts. Whole grains retain their bran and germ, offering fiber and nutrients that promote digestive health.

2. Greek Yogurt for Sour Cream: Swap sour cream with Greek yogurt for creaminess and tanginess in dishes like dips, dressings, and baked goods. You'll enjoy added protein and probiotics.

3. *Avocado for Butter:* In baking and spreads, use mashed avocado as a butter substitute. It brings healthy fats and a creamy texture to your recipes.

4. *Applesauce for Oil:* Applesauce can replace oil in baking recipes, reducing the overall fat content while maintaining moisture and sweetness.

5. *Nut Flours for Regular Flour:* Experiment with almond flour, coconut flour, or oat flour as alternatives to refined wheat flour. These options are gluten-free and add nutty flavors.

6. *Lean Proteins for Fatty Meats:* Opt for lean meats like chicken, turkey, and fish instead of fatty cuts. These options are lower in saturated fats and calories.

Exploring Flavorful Substitutions
1. *Herbs and Spices for Salt:* Use herbs, spices, and citrus to enhance flavor instead of excessive salt. This adds depth to your dishes while reducing sodium intake.

2. *Natural Sweeteners for White Sugar:* Swap white sugar with natural sweeteners like honey, maple syrup, or stevia. They bring sweetness with added nutrients.

3. *Nutritional Yeast for Cheese:* Nutritional yeast adds a cheesy flavor to dishes without the saturated fat found in traditional cheese.

Navigating Allergies and Dietary Preferences
Ingredient swaps also cater to dietary restrictions and preferences. For dairy-free alternatives, consider plant-based milk, such as almond or oat milk. To accommodate gluten sensitivities, experiment with gluten-free flours or grains like quinoa and buckwheat.

Empowering Your Culinary Adventure
Embarking on a healthier culinary journey is an adventure that unveils a world of possibilities. Ingredient swaps allow you to honor your taste buds and prioritize your well-being. As you explore new flavors and textures, you'll discover that the art of substitution not only transforms your dishes but also enhances your appreciation for the nourishing power of food. So, embrace the joy of experimenting, and let ingredient swaps be your compass as you create dishes that uplift both your palate and your health.

Achieving Balance in Every Meal and Snack

Creating a sense of balance in your meals and snacks is the cornerstone of a healthful and satisfying eating routine. In this section, we'll delve into the art of crafting balanced plates and snacks that provide the nourishment your body craves while delighting your senses. Whether it's breakfast, lunch, dinner, or a quick snack, finding equilibrium in your choices allows you to savor both the flavors of your food and the wellness it brings.

Achieving balance in your meals means assembling a combination of nutrients that work in harmony to support your energy, digestion, and overall well-being. Here's how you can create balanced plates that leave you both satisfied and nourished:

1. Incorporate All Food Groups: Each meal should include a variety of food groups: lean proteins, whole grains, colorful vegetables, and healthy fats. This ensures a spectrum of nutrients that your body needs to function optimally.

2. Protein Power: Prioritize protein sources like lean meats, poultry, fish, beans, lentils, tofu, and Greek yogurt. Protein stabilizes blood sugar, provides satiety, and supports muscle health.

3. *Whole Grain Goodness:* Choose whole grains like quinoa, brown rice, whole wheat pasta, and oats. These provide complex carbohydrates and fiber that release energy slowly.

4. *Vibrant Vegetables:* Fill half your plate with non-starchy vegetables, such as leafy greens, bell peppers, and carrots. These provide vitamins, minerals, and fiber.

5. *Healthy Fats:* Include sources of healthy fats like avocados, nuts, seeds, and olive oil. These fats are essential for nutrient absorption and overall well-being.

Creating Balanced Snacks: Nourishment Between Meals

Balanced snacks are your secret weapon for maintaining energy levels and preventing excessive hunger between meals. Here's how you can curate snacks that keep you on track:

1. *Pair Protein with Fiber:* Combine protein-rich foods with high-fiber options. For instance, pair Greek yogurt with berries or apple slices with nut butter. This combination provides sustained energy and satiety.

2. *Portion Control:* Even for snacks, portion control is key. Use small bowls or containers to prevent mindless overeating.

3. *Nutrient Variety:* Choose snacks that offer a mix of nutrients. For example, hummus with carrot sticks provides protein, healthy fats, and vitamins.

4. *Hydrate Wisely:* Opt for hydrating snacks like cucumber slices or watermelon cubes. Hydration supports digestion and keeps you feeling refreshed.

The Joy of Mindful Eating

Achieving balance in every meal and snack is an invitation to savor the joy of mindful eating. By selecting a diverse array of foods and nourishing your body with intention, you're nurturing yourself holistically. This practice not only honors your taste buds but also supports your energy levels, mood, and overall vitality.

So, whether you're crafting a colorful salad for lunch, enjoying a balanced dinner with loved ones, or savoring a satisfying snack on the go, let the essence of balance be your guiding principle. In doing so, you're not just creating meals and snacks; you're nurturing a sense of harmony that resonates throughout your well-being – an exquisite symphony of flavors and nourishment that leaves you feeling nourished, vibrant, and truly satisfied.

Chapter 13

Cooking for Picky Eaters

Clever Strategies to Sneak in More Veggies

Navigating mealtime with picky eaters can be a culinary adventure all its own. However, with a dash of creativity and a sprinkle of ingenuity, you can transform meals into a delightful experience that encourages the consumption of nutritious vegetables. In this section, we'll uncover strategies to triumph over picky palates and sneak in those essential veggies without compromising on taste or enjoyment.

Picky eaters often have preferences that lean towards familiar tastes and textures. The challenge lies in introducing new flavors, especially when it comes to vegetables. But fret not; with these clever strategies, you can pave the way for a more veggie-friendly dining experience:

*1. **Blend and Mix:*** Incorporate vegetables into smoothies, sauces, and soups. Blending vegetables like spinach, carrots, and cauliflower into smoothies or adding pureed veggies to pasta sauces can introduce their goodness in subtle ways.

*2. **Creative Disguises:*** Play with shapes and sizes to make veggies more appealing. Create fun vegetable kebabs, vegetable "fries," or veggie-packed mini muffins. The element of novelty can pique curiosity.

*3. **Sensory Exploration:*** Encourage kids to touch, smell, and interact with vegetables before eating. This sensory engagement can make them more open to trying new foods.

*4. **Dip Delights:*** Pair veggies with flavorful dips like hummus, yogurt-based dressings, or nut butter. The dip can provide a familiar taste that eases them into trying new textures.

*5. **Cooking Collaborations:*** Involve picky eaters in meal preparation. Kids are more likely to eat what they've helped create, fostering a sense of ownership and curiosity.

Veggies in Familiar Favorites: A Flavorful Transformation

Transforming beloved dishes into veggie-rich creations is a clever way to introduce vegetables without the resistance. Here are some ideas:

1. *Sneaky Sauces:* Puree vegetables like zucchini, carrots, or bell peppers and add them to pasta sauces, stews, and casseroles. The added depth of flavor can be a delightful surprise.

2. *Veggie Pizzas:* Top pizzas with a rainbow of vegetables, from bell peppers to cherry tomatoes, mushrooms, and spinach. Kids can even join in the pizza-making process.

3. *Veggie Noodles:* Swap regular pasta with zucchini noodles (zoodles) or sweet potato noodles for a colorful and nutrient-packed twist.

4. *Cauliflower Magic:* Transform cauliflower into "rice," "mashed potatoes," or even "buffalo wings." The mild flavor of cauliflower makes it an excellent canvas for creativity.

5. *Stuffed Creations:* Fill stuffed peppers or mushrooms with a flavorful mixture of vegetables and protein. These tasty packages can make veggies feel like a delicious adventure.

Cultivating a Positive Veggie Experience

Cooking for picky eaters is an opportunity to create a positive relationship with food, including vegetables. By incorporating these strategies, you're fostering a sense of curiosity and exploration that can lead to a more varied and nutritious diet. Remember, it's a gradual process; be patient and celebrate even small victories.

So, whether you're crafting veggie-packed burgers, presenting vegetable "hidden treasures," or transforming familiar dishes into nutrient-rich delights, let these strategies guide your culinary journey. As you gradually introduce veggies with creativity and a touch of playfulness, you're not just nourishing growing bodies; you're cultivating a love for food that's rich in color, taste, and healthful abundance.

Kid-Approved Healthy Swaps for Happy Plates

Nurturing the well-being of your little ones doesn't mean sacrificing the joy of delicious meals. In fact, with a sprinkle of creativity and a dash of innovation, you can transform their plates into vibrant feasts that celebrate health and happiness. In this section, we'll dive into kid-approved healthy swaps that not only nourish growing bodies but also put smiles on their faces.

Healthy swaps are the secret ingredient to turning everyday meals into adventures of flavor and nutrition. By replacing certain ingredients with more wholesome options, you can create a balanced harmony between taste and well-being. Here's how you can make your kids' plates a canvas of color and joy:

1. Whole Grain Wonders:
Trade white bread for whole wheat or whole grain versions. Switch out regular pasta with whole wheat or legume-based pasta. These swaps introduce more fiber and nutrients to their diets.

2. Colorful Veggie Delights:
Enhance the vibrancy of their meals by adding a rainbow of vegetables. Sneak grated carrots into muffins, blend

spinach into smoothies, and stuff bell peppers with a medley of goodness.

3. Fruitful Sweetness:
Opt for natural sweetness by using mashed bananas, unsweetened applesauce, or dates in recipes. These alternatives add a touch of sweetness while bringing in essential nutrients.

4. Protein-Packed Twists:
Replace processed meats with lean protein sources like chicken, turkey, beans, lentils, or tofu. Create delightful wraps, skewers, and stir-fries that tickle their taste buds.

5. Dairy Dazzle:
Choose low-fat or Greek yogurt instead of sugary flavored yogurts. Swap whole milk with skim or plant-based alternatives for their cereal and recipes.

6. Wholesome Snacking:
Trade store-bought chips with air-popped popcorn, veggie sticks, or whole grain crackers paired with nut butter or hummus for dipping.

7. Nutrient-Rich Sweets:
Bake treats with whole grains, natural sweeteners, and added fruits. Think banana bread, oatmeal cookies, or even chia seed pudding.

8. *Hydration Heroes:*
Encourage water consumption by offering infused water with slices of fruits or cucumbers. Limit sugary drinks and opt for real fruit juices in moderation.

Culinary Adventures with Joyful Swaps
Healthy swaps are like secret treasures that turn meals into exciting culinary adventures. By infusing nutrient-rich ingredients, you're not just nurturing their bodies; you're nurturing a positive relationship with food. As you embark on this journey of flavor and wholesome joy, remember to keep an open mind, involve your kids in the process, and celebrate the wins, no matter how small.

So, whether you're preparing a veggie-loaded pizza, crafting energy-boosting snacks, or serving up a plate that's a vibrant tapestry of colors, let these kid-approved healthy swaps be your guide. In each bite, your little ones will experience a symphony of taste, nourishment, and delight that forms the foundation for a future filled with well-being and happiness.

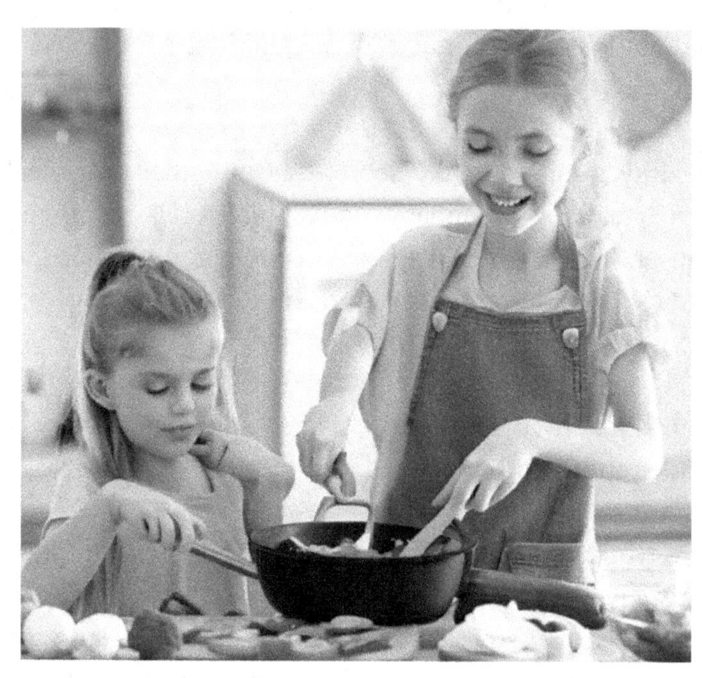

Chapter 14

Weekly Meal Plans

Sample Meal Plan 1: Effortless Weekday Dinners

Life's busy rhythm calls for meal planning that's both convenient and satisfying. Sample Meal Plan 1 is designed to make your weekday evenings a breeze by offering a delightful array of dinners that require minimal effort without compromising on flavor or nutrition. With a mix of wholesome ingredients and simple preparation, you'll savor delicious meals that bring ease to your evenings.

Day 1: Honey Glazed Salmon with Roasted Veggies
- Honey-glazed salmon fillets, baked to perfection
- A side of roasted mixed vegetables (bell peppers, broccoli, and carrots) drizzled with olive oil and a touch of seasoning

Day 2: One-Pan Chicken and Veggie Stir-Fry
- Quick and easy chicken stir-fry with an assortment of colorful bell peppers, snap peas, and carrots
- Served over a bed of fluffy brown rice or quinoa

Day 3: Veggie-Packed Pasta Primavera
- Whole wheat pasta adorned with a medley of sautéed zucchini, cherry tomatoes, spinach, and garlic
- Tossed in a light olive oil and lemon juice dressing, topped with grated Parmesan

Day 4: Black Bean and Sweet Potato Tacos
- Hearty black bean and sweet potato filling seasoned with cumin and chili powder
- Assembled into soft tortillas, topped with diced avocado, salsa, and a dollop of Greek yogurt

Day 5: Quinoa Bowl with Mediterranean Flair
- Nutrient-rich quinoa topped with a colorful combination of chopped cucumber, cherry tomatoes, red onion, kalamata olives, and crumbled feta cheese
- Drizzled with a zesty lemon vinaigrette

Day 6: Grilled Chicken Caesar Salad
- Grilled chicken breast served on a bed of fresh romaine lettuce
- Tossed with whole wheat croutons, grated Parmesan, and a light Caesar dressing

Day 7: Veggie and Brown Rice Stir-Fry
- Wholesome brown rice stir-fry featuring an assortment of your favorite vegetables (broccoli, carrots, bell peppers, and snap peas)
- Flavored with soy sauce and a touch of sesame oil

Effortless Delights at Your Fingertips
Sample Meal Plan 1 takes the guesswork out of weekday dinners, offering you a diverse range of flavors and ingredients that come together with minimal fuss. Each dish celebrates the beauty of simplicity while ensuring you enjoy a balanced and nourishing meal. With this plan in hand, you're not just creating dinners; you're crafting moments of culinary delight that allow you to savor the joy of a well-prepared meal without the stress of elaborate cooking. Cheers to effortless evenings filled with deliciousness and wholesome satisfaction!

Sample Meal Plan 2: Quick Breakfasts and On-the-Go Lunches

Life's fast-paced rhythm demands meal planning that fits seamlessly into busy mornings and bustling afternoons. Sample Meal Plan 2 is your solution, offering a delightful array of quick breakfasts and on-the-go lunches that provide nourishment without compromising on taste or convenience. With a mix of energy-boosting breakfasts and portable lunches, you'll savor satisfying meals that fuel your day.

Day 1: Energizing Breakfast Smoothie
- Blend a nutritious smoothie with spinach, banana, frozen berries, Greek yogurt, and a splash of almond milk
- Perfect for a quick breakfast on busy mornings

Day 2: Overnight Oats On-the-Go
- Prepare overnight oats by combining rolled oats, chia seeds, almond milk, and a drizzle of honey
- Top with sliced almonds and fresh berries for a delicious portable breakfast

Day 3: Classic Avocado Toast
- Spread smashed avocado on whole grain toast
- Top with sliced tomato, a sprinkle of red pepper flakes, and a drizzle of olive oil

Day 4: Veggie Wrap with Hummus
- Assemble a whole wheat wrap filled with hummus, sliced cucumbers, bell peppers, and baby spinach
- Perfect for an on-the-go lunch

Day 5: Quinoa Salad Jar
- Layer a mason jar with cooked quinoa, black beans, corn, diced red onion, and mixed greens
- Top with a zesty vinaigrette for a convenient and nutritious lunch

Day 6: Nut Butter and Banana Sandwich
- Spread your favorite nut butter on whole grain bread
- Add sliced banana and a sprinkle of cinnamon for a quick and satisfying breakfast or lunch

Day 7: Greek Yogurt Parfait To-Go
- Layer a portable container with Greek yogurt, granola, and mixed berries
- Enjoy a creamy and crunchy on-the-go snack or breakfast

Efficiency Meets Flavorful Nutrition

Sample Meal Plan 2 simplifies your breakfast and lunch routines, providing you with quick yet delicious options that seamlessly fit into your busy schedule. Each meal celebrates the art of simplicity while ensuring you receive the nutrients and energy you need. With this plan at your fingertips, you're not just planning meals; you're crafting moments of nourishment and satisfaction that effortlessly align with your fast-paced lifestyle. Here's to starting your day with vitality and tackling afternoons with sustained energy, all while enjoying the delights of well-prepared meals.

Sample Meal Plan 3: Enjoyable Family Weekend Feasts

Weekends are an opportunity to gather, savor, and relish in the joy of shared meals with your loved ones. Sample Meal Plan 3 is designed to make your family weekends memorable by offering a delectable array of dishes that celebrate togetherness and the pleasures of indulgence. With a mix of comforting classics and exciting flavors, you'll create feasts that warm your hearts and nourish your souls.

Day 1: Saturday Breakfast Spread

Pancake Party: Stack fluffy pancakes with a variety of toppings like fresh berries, sliced bananas, chopped nuts, and a drizzle of maple syrup.

Scrambled Eggs with a Twist: Add sautéed spinach, diced tomatoes, and shredded cheddar cheese to scrambled eggs for a flavorful morning delight.

Day 2: Hearty Sunday Brunch

- Omelette Extravaganza: Set up an omelette bar with a range of fillings such as diced ham, bell peppers, onions, mushrooms, and shredded cheese.
- Roasted Potatoes: Serve crispy roasted potatoes seasoned with rosemary and garlic alongside.

Day 3: Comforting Sunday Dinner
Slow-Cooked Pot Roast: Prepare a tender pot roast with root vegetables like carrots, potatoes, and onions, slow-cooked in savory broth.
Creamy Mashed Potatoes: Whip up creamy mashed potatoes for a comforting side.
Steamed Green Beans: Steam fresh green beans and toss with a touch of butter and slivered almonds.

Day 4: Wholesome Saturday Lunch
Build-Your-Own Salad: Create a vibrant salad bar with mixed greens, an array of chopped veggies, grilled chicken or tofu, and an assortment of dressings.
Freshly Baked Bread: Serve warm, crusty bread for a satisfying accompaniment.

Day 5: Outdoor Sunday BBQ
Grilled Burgers and Hot Dogs: Fire up the grill for classic burgers and hot dogs with an array of condiments and toppings.
Grilled Corn on the Cob: Grill corn on the cob with a brushed-on garlic butter for smoky sweetness.

Day 6: Family Pizza Night
Pizza Creation Station: Set out pizza dough, sauce, cheese, and an array of toppings so each family member can build their own personalized pizza.

Salad Bar: Accompany pizzas with a DIY salad bar featuring fresh greens, veggies, and a variety of dressings.

Day 7: Sunday Evening Roast Chicken

- Roast Chicken: Prepare a succulent roast chicken with a blend of herbs, lemon, and garlic, resulting in tender and flavorful meat.
- Quinoa Pilaf: Serve alongside a fragrant quinoa pilaf with sautéed onions, dried cranberries, and toasted almonds.

Creating Treasured Family Moments

Sample Meal Plan 3 transforms family weekends into culinary celebrations that bring loved ones closer and create lasting memories. Each meal embraces the spirit of togetherness while offering a symphony of flavors and textures. With this plan in hand, you're not just cooking; you're crafting moments that celebrate the beauty of sharing meals, laughter, and joy. Here's to weekends filled with delicious feasts that nourish both body and soul, and to creating cherished memories that will be savored for years to come.

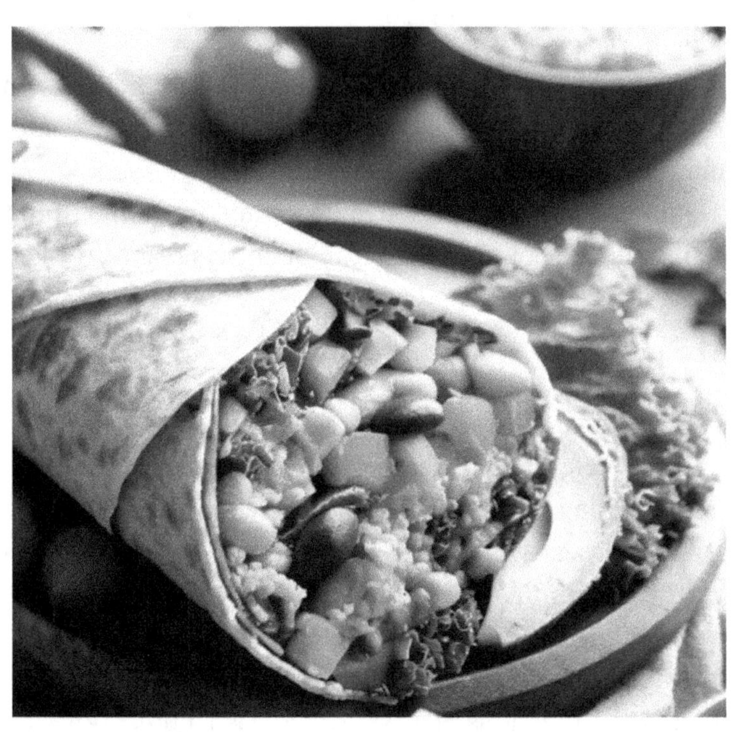

Appendix

Nutritional Insights and Serving Guidelines

The appendix serves as a valuable resource that enhances your understanding of the nutritional aspects of cooking, providing you with insights and guidelines to make informed and health-conscious choices. By delving into this section, you'll gain a deeper appreciation for the role of nutrition in your culinary journey and how it contributes to overall well-being.

Understanding Nutritional Components: Building Blocks of Health
Nutrition forms the foundation of a balanced and healthy lifestyle. In this section, you'll explore the essential components that make up your meals:

Macronutrients: Discover the significance of carbohydrates, proteins, and fats in fueling your body and maintaining its functions. Learn how to incorporate a balanced ratio of these macronutrients into your meals to support energy levels and growth.

Micronutrients: Delve into the world of vitamins and minerals, understanding their roles in boosting immunity, supporting bone health, and facilitating various bodily processes. Discover which foods are rich sources of essential micronutrients.

Portion Control and Serving Guidelines: A Balance of Quality and Quantity

Achieving a balance between quality and quantity is crucial for maintaining a healthful diet. This section offers insights into portion control and appropriate serving sizes:

Portion Awareness: Gain an understanding of portion distortion and how it can lead to overconsumption. Learn strategies to become more mindful of portion sizes, ensuring you enjoy meals in moderation.

Visual Cues: Discover visual cues that can help you estimate appropriate serving sizes without the need for measuring tools. Learn to use your hand, plate, and other indicators to gauge portion proportions.

Balanced Plates: Explore the concept of balanced meals, where vegetables, proteins, carbohydrates, and healthy fats come together harmoniously. Acquire the knowledge to construct plates that provide sustained energy and a variety of nutrients.

Tailoring Nutrition to Individual Needs:
Everyone's nutritional needs are unique. This section helps you consider factors such as age, activity level, and health goals when planning meals:

Caloric Intake: Learn how to estimate your daily caloric needs based on factors like age, gender, and activity level. This knowledge allows you to adjust portion sizes and meal composition to align with your goals.

Special Dietary Considerations: Discover how to tailor your meals to accommodate dietary restrictions, whether it's for weight management, managing health conditions, or following a specific eating plan.

Empowerment Through Nutritional Knowledge:
As you explore this section, you'll gain valuable insights that empower you to make conscious choices about what you eat. Armed with a deeper understanding of nutritional components, portion control, and individual needs, you'll approach your culinary creations with a newfound awareness of how they contribute to your overall health and well-being. With each meal you prepare, you're not just satisfying your taste buds; you're nurturing your body and embracing the potential for a vibrant and nourished life.

Glossary of Essential Cooking Terminology

The art of cooking is woven with a rich tapestry of terms that describe techniques, tools, ingredients, and processes. This glossary is your gateway to understanding and mastering the language of the kitchen. Whether you're a culinary enthusiast or a seasoned chef, this comprehensive collection of essential cooking terminology will empower you to navigate recipes with confidence and finesse, elevating your cooking skills to new heights.

Al Dente: An Italian term referring to pasta that is cooked to a firm yet tender texture, offering a slight resistance when bitten.

Bain-Marie: A gentle method of heating or melting ingredients by placing a container within another container filled with water, ensuring gradual and even heat distribution.

Deglaze: To loosen and dissolve flavorful browned bits (fond) that stick to the bottom of a pan after sautéing or searing, often done by adding liquid such as wine or broth and stirring to incorporate those flavors into a sauce.

Emulsify: The process of combining two immiscible liquids, such as oil and vinegar, into a smooth and cohesive mixture through vigorous whisking or blending.

Fold: A gentle mixing technique used to combine delicate ingredients, where one mixture is incorporated into another using a spatula in a gentle lifting and folding motion.

Julienne: To cut vegetables, fruits, or other ingredients into thin, matchstick-like strips, often used for garnishes or stir-fries.

Knead: The process of working dough with hands to develop gluten, creating elasticity and structure in bread or pasta.

Mise en Place: A French term meaning "everything in its place." It refers to the practice of prepping and organizing all ingredients before starting to cook, ensuring a smooth and efficient cooking process.

Pâte à Choux: A versatile dough used to make pastries like éclairs and cream puffs, achieved by cooking flour, butter, water, and eggs together.

Render: To melt and separate fat from meat or other food items by cooking over low heat, producing flavorful fat that can be used for cooking or sautéing.

Sauté: A quick cooking method that involves cooking food rapidly in a small amount of oil or fat over high heat, often stirring or tossing to evenly cook and develop flavors.

Tangy: A flavor profile characterized by a sharp, slightly sour taste, often associated with ingredients like citrus fruits, vinegar, or fermented foods.

Umami: Often referred to as the fifth taste, umami is a savory flavor that enhances the overall taste experience, found in ingredients like tomatoes, mushrooms, soy sauce, and aged cheeses.

Velveting: A technique used in Chinese cuisine to tenderize and coat proteins by marinating them in a mixture of cornstarch and egg white before cooking.

Whisk: A kitchen tool used to combine ingredients, incorporating air and creating a smooth texture through a rapid back-and-forth motion.

Zest: The outermost layer of citrus peel, often used to add bright, aromatic flavor to dishes by grating or peeling the colored part of the peel.

Unlocking the Culinary Language:

As you immerse yourself in the world of cooking, this glossary acts as your guide to understanding the intricate vocabulary that enriches your culinary creations. Each term you embrace brings you one step closer to cooking with precision, creativity, and the finesse of a seasoned chef. Whether you're braising, blanching, or browning, each word adds depth to your culinary language and empowers you to craft dishes that tell a story of taste, technique, and passion.